Face Creams, Hair Rinses, and Body Lotions

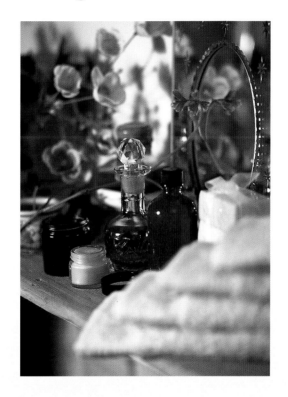

how to make your own organic cosmetics

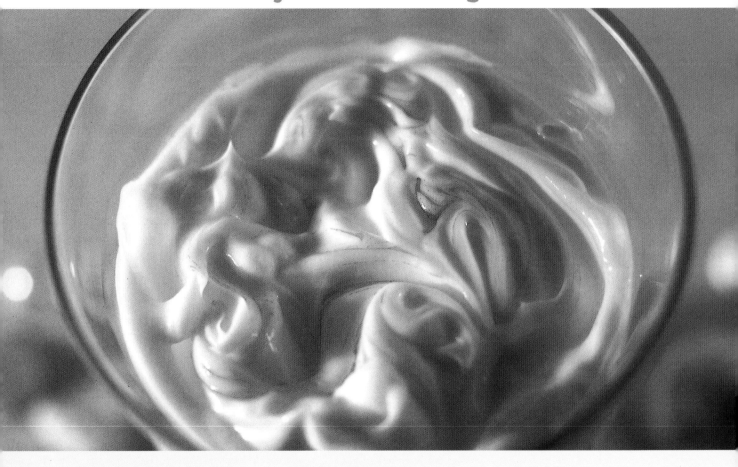

GILL FARRER-HALLS

Face Creams, Hair Rinses, and Body Lotions:

Recipes for Natural Beauty

GLOUCESTER MASSACHUSETTS

QUARRY BOOKS

First published in the United States of America by
Quarry Books, an imprint of
Rockport Publishers, Inc.
33 Commercial Street
Gloucester, Massachusetts 01930-5089
Telephone: (978) 282-9590
Fax: (978) 283-2742
www.rockpub.com

Library of Congress Cataloging-in-Publication Data
Farrer-Halls, Gill.
    Face creams, hair rinses, and body lotions : recipes for natural beauty
/ Gill Farrer-Halls
        p.   cm. — (How to make your own organic cosmetics)
    ISBN 1-59253-108-3 (pbk.)
    1. Herbal cosmetics. 2. Beauty, Personal. 3. Women—Health and hygiene
I. Title. II. Series.
RA778.F374 2004
668'.55—dc22   2004006843
                                                                      CIP

ISBN 1-59253-108-3

10 9 8 7 6 5 4 3 2 1

Design: Toby Matthews, toby.matthews@ntlworld.com
Photography: Robin Bath
Book packaged by Angie Patchell, atpatchell@ntlworld.com

Printed in China

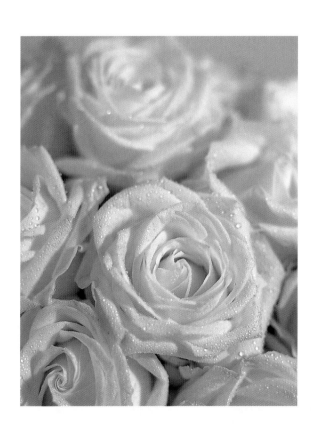

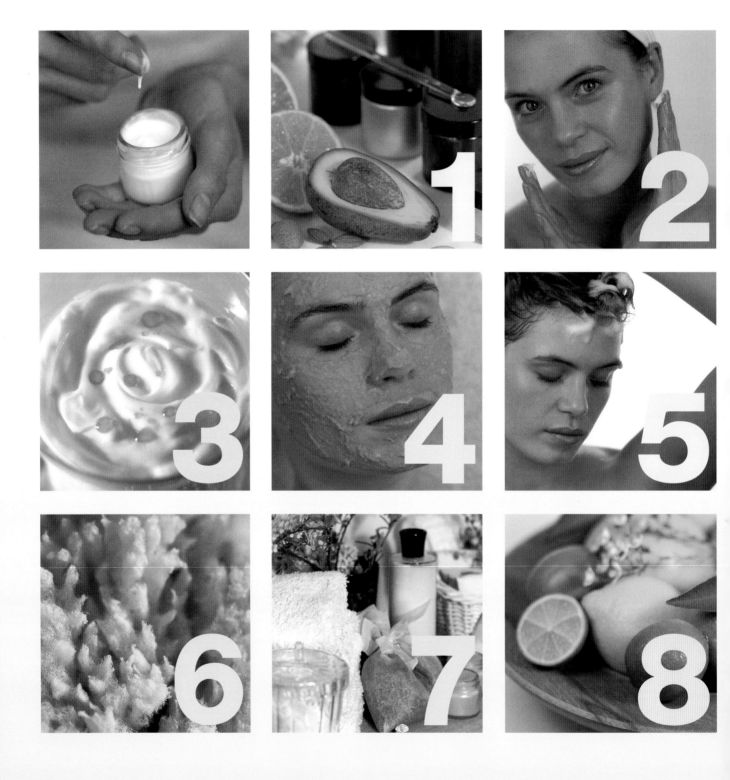

Contents

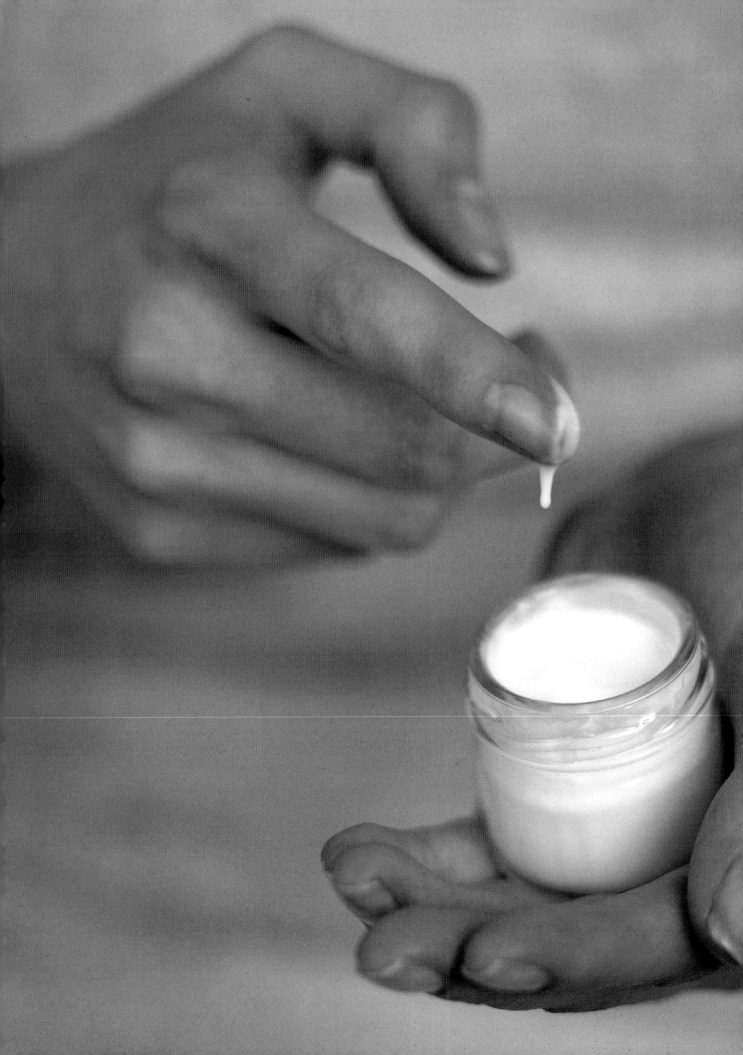

Introduction

"It is relatively easy to make simple creams, lotions, and aromatic waters for the skin at home using essential oils, beeswax, cocoa butter, and flower waters...."

–Patricia Davis, *author and aromatherapist*

Introduction

The skin is more important than just the wrapping around our body. It is, in fact, the body's largest organ, and it plays several roles in the healthy functioning of the whole body. One of the skin's major characteristics is that it is semipermeable. This means that certain substances can pass through the skin while others are simultaneously blocked. Thus, the skin both nourishes and protects the body. To illustrate, many toxins are sweated out through the skin and many nutrients are absorbed into the body through the skin. Bacteria are prevented entry to the body, and valuable bodily fluids are contained.

This knowledge emphasizes that what you put on your face and skin is as important as what you eat. Or, in other words, natural, organic cosmetics are as good for you as natural, organic foods. Some of the ingredients used to make your own cosmetics can be found in the kitchen, so—theoretically of course!—some of your homemade products are good enough to eat. Other ingredients can be sourced from organic cosmetics suppliers. The recipes in this book use only plant-based ingredients that are not tested on animals, so in keeping with the organics philosophy, you can have beauty without cruelty.

Effective skin care is necessary to keep the skin supple and in good condition so that it both looks beautiful and fulfills its functions. Using natural, organic substances such as flower waters, essential oils, honey, fruits, and so forth in homemade cosmetics can provide a wide range of skin treatments for all the different types of skin. The recipes included here range from simple additions to base creams and lotions to actually cooking up your own face and hand creams. No matter which recipes appeal to you, you can trust that your own homemade lotions and potions are natural and healthy. They also tend to work out to be cheaper than store-bought cosmetics, so you can afford to experiment and try out new skin care ideas.

Many of the ingredients and techniques for making your own creams have been in use for thousands of years. They are known from long experience to be effective, safe, and beneficial to your skin. For example, honey, almond oil, and lemon have all been used extensively over the

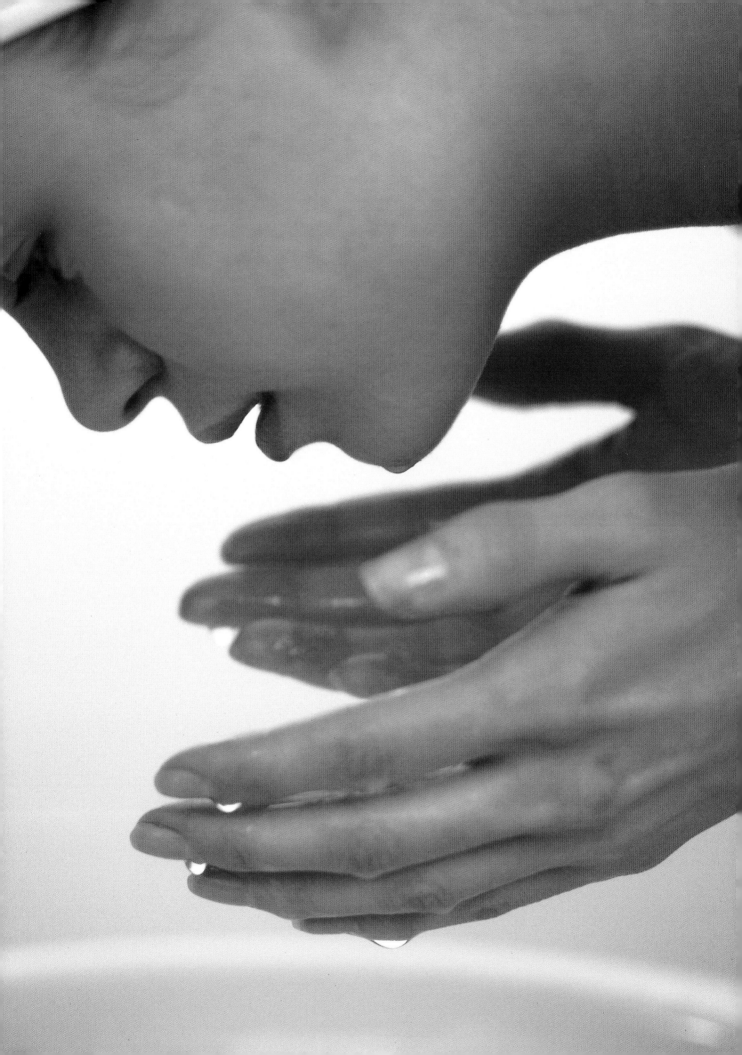

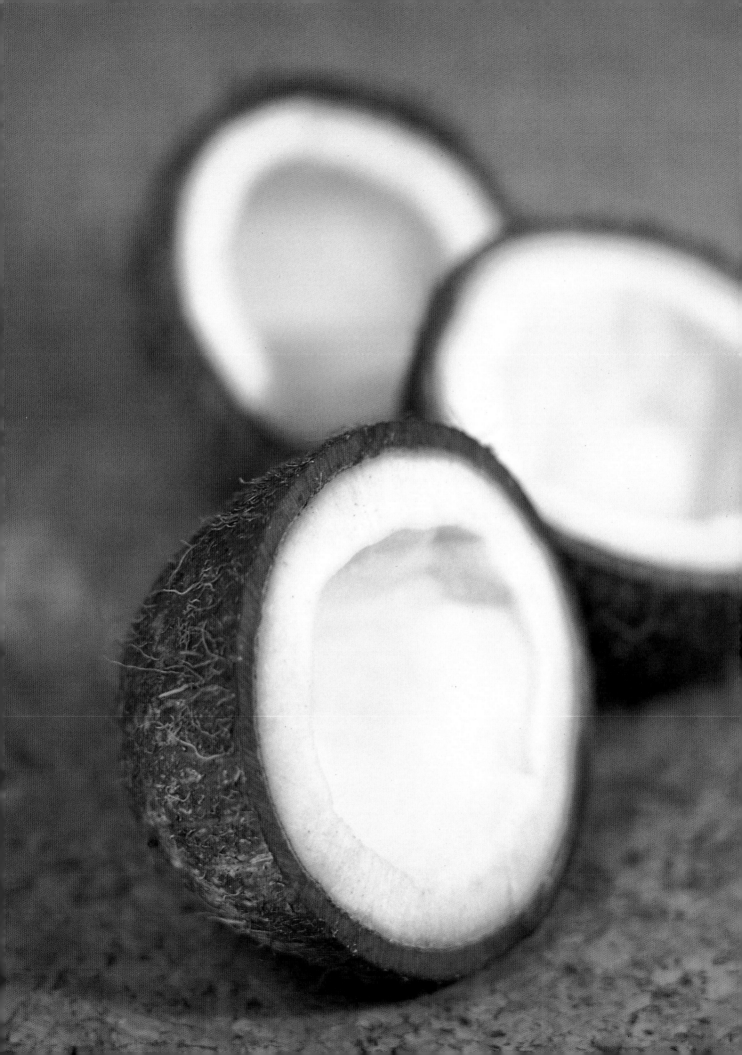

centuries. Honey is effective for healing and softening skin, and has been used successfully to treat minor burns. Lemon is a gentle skin bleach, helping fade freckles and age spots, and it brightens hair when used as a hair rinse. The soothing, moisturising, and nourishing effects of almond oil are well known skin care secrets that have been passed on orally between generations of women.

Essential oils have also been used consistently in skin care and beauty treatments almost since the time of their discovery. There are many benefits in using natural and organic essential oils in your home made skin creams, lotions, and potions. Essential oils are proven to speed up the removal of old skin cells and to stimulate the growth of new skin cells. They reduce inflammation and regulate the production of sebum, and, above all, their wonderful scents are calming and soothing, reducing stress and aiding relaxation. Certain essential oils have a rejuvenating effect on the skin and can help to keep you looking and feeling youthful and beautiful.

Some of the more modern store-bought concoctions tend to use chemicals, and animal and mineral substances. Not all of these are harmless to ourselves, to animals, or our environment, so the recipes here suggest using only organic and plant-based ingredients. Using organic and natural plant-based cosmetics means that your preparations are safer, more efficacious, more environmentally friendly, and generate an overall sense of well being. When buying lotion and cream bases, you can check whether these are made using organic, plant-based ingredients.

The included recipes range from the incredibly simple right up to blending sophisticated and complex skin creams. This means you can design your skin care cosmetics to exactly match your skin type and condition. You can start by simply stirring in essential oils to cream and lotion bases. Once you have experimented with these recipes and feel confident, you can move on to creating skin creams using flower waters, beeswax, essential oils, and other natural and organic ingredients.

In addition to recipes for face and hand creams and body lotions, there are also recipes for making shampoos, conditioners, and rejuvenating hair treatments, as well as lip balms, skin toners, deodorants, aftershaves, and face masks. This provides a comprehensive range of natural cosmetics to make, use, and enjoy. You can also trust that they are good for you and the environment.

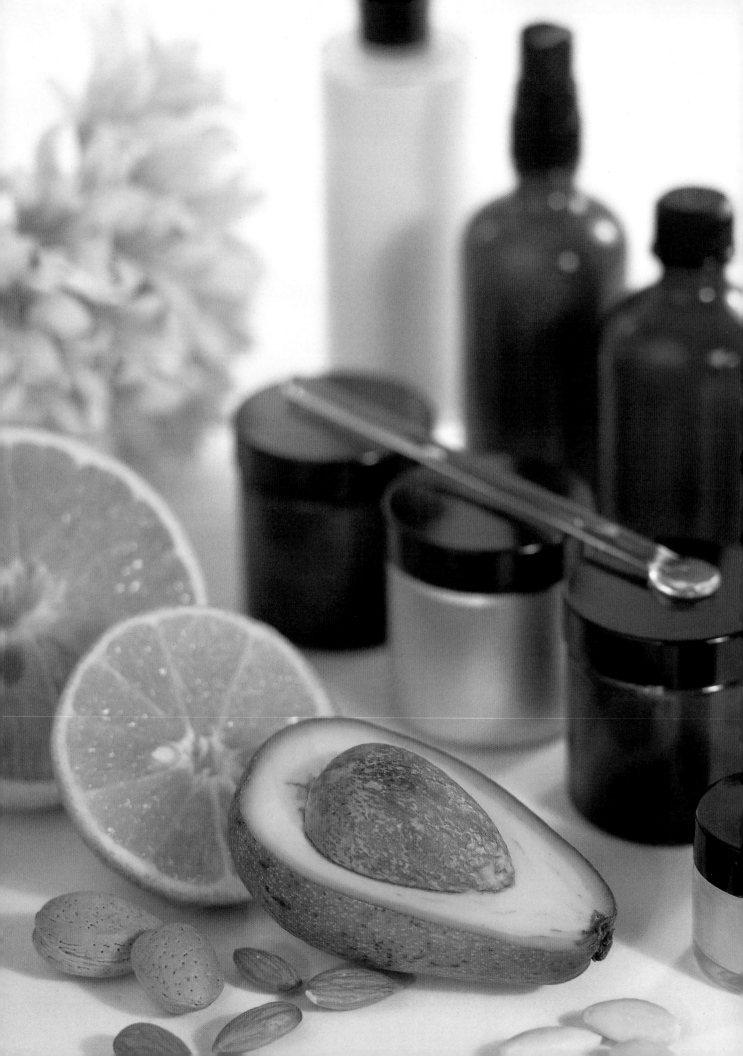

Chapter One

Ingredients and Equipment

"Common sense and caution should go hand in hand when deciding on the choice of oils and strength of dilution."
                    —Patricia Davis, *author and aromatherapist*

Essential Oils and How to Use Them Safely

Essential oils are used extensively in the hand-made cosmetics in this book. The oils bring healing and protective skin-care qualities to all the products, as well as enhancing these products with their delightful fragrances. Essential oils are highly concentrated, as can be seen by the fact that it takes thousands of jasmine petals to produce a single drop of jasmine. This potency must be respected, and thus how you handle essential oils is important. Because essential oils are powerful and concentrated, they can be toxic if used incorrectly. However, if you handle oils carefully and follow these simple guidelines, they are quite safe for all your homemade cosmetics.

- Never take essential oils orally. It is illegal for even a qualified aromatherapist to suggest this. Avoid all contact with the mouth and eyes.

- Some essential oils can cause skin irritation if they are applied undiluted to the skin, therefore this is not recommended. Apply only properly diluted essential oils to the skin.

- The A–Z of Essential Oils section on page 18 indicates which oils might cause skin irritation for those with sensitive skin. Occasionally, a slight redness or itchiness might occur from using these or any other essential oil. If this happens, apply some base cream or base oil, such as almond oil, to the affected area and place a cold, wet cloth on the affected area until the redness or itchiness disappears.

- Do not be tempted to increase the amount of essential oils used in the recipes and follow the instructions carefully.

- If you accidentally splash a drop of essential oil in your eye, use a small amount of base oil to dilute the essential oil, absorb this with a soft cloth, then rinse the eyes with cold water.

- A few essential oils, such as bergamot, lemon, and the other citrus oils, are phototoxic. This means they might cause skin discoloration when exposed to bright sunlight, though once incorporated into skin-care products they are diluted and quite safe. However, it is best to avoid using face creams and body lotions containing bergamot and other citrus oils if the weather is hot and sunny.

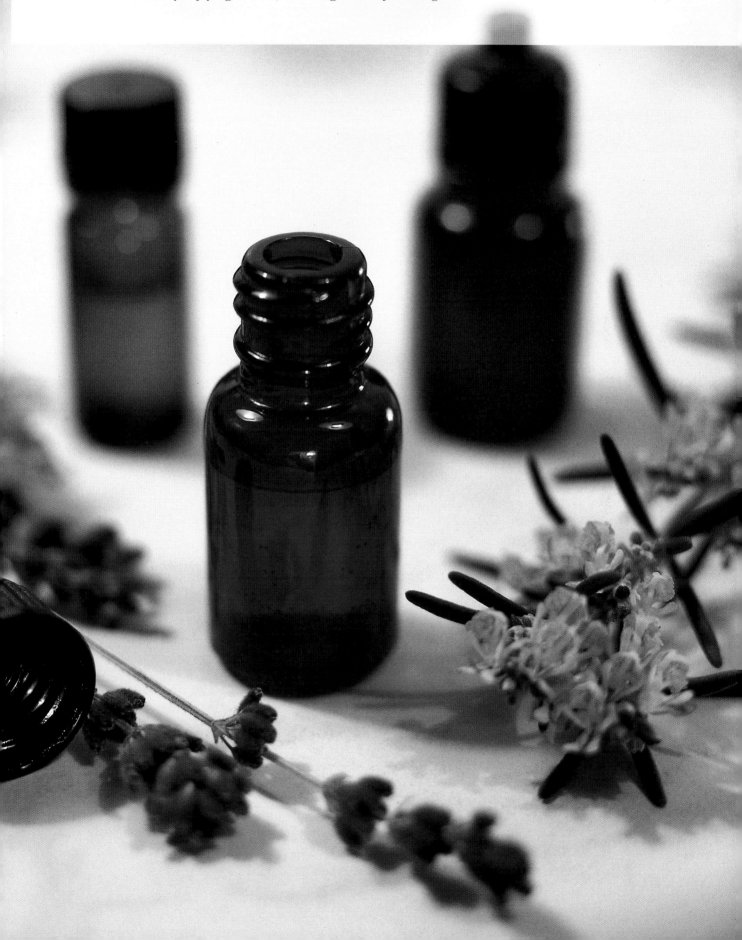

Tip: *When you finish an essential oil and the bottle is empty, reward yourself with a beaufully fragranced, relaxing bath by rinsing it out in the water.*

A–Z of Essential Oils

Essential oils are nature's gift. They are distilled from the naturally occurring essences in aromatic plants. Many essential oils are distilled from organically grown plants, and these are the best to use in making your cosmetics. Below is a list of the main essential oils used in the recipes, together with a description of their fragrances and qualities. A "P" indicates the oil should not to be used during pregnancy. An "S" indicates a possibility of skin irritation for people with sensitive skin.

Bergamot
(citrus bergamia)

Bergamot is grown in Italy, and is the finest of the citrus oils. It has fresh, lemon top notes and floral, balsamic undertones. *S*

Chamomile Roman/Chamomile German
(anthemis nobilis/matricaria chamomilla)

Chamomile has a calming, soothing effect on the skin. The fragrance has hints of apple among bitter, herbaceous undertones and warm, flowery top notes. *P*

Frankincense
(boswellia carteri)

Frankincense was used in the embalming of bodies in ancient Egypt and has antiaging properties. It combines citrus, turpentine top notes with undertones of camphor and balsamic wood smoke.

Geranium
(pelargonium gravolens)

Geranium helps regulate sebum production in the skin and is generally balancing. It has light, green top notes and soft, rosy, floral undertones. *P*

Jasmine
(jasminum officinale)

Jasmine combines a powerful, heady fragrance with excellent skin care properties, especially for dry, sensitive skin. Jasmine has sweet, floral, exotic top notes and heady, warm, honeyed undertones. *P*

Lavender
(lavandula vera)

Lavender is the most popular and widely used essential oil, and has soothing, anti-inflammatory properties. Lavender's calming qualities helps promote sleep. It has clean, fresh, floral top notes and subtle, green, herbaceous undertones.

Lemon
(citrus limon)

The fresh smell of lemon is a familiar one. Lemon is also an astringent, making it useful for greasy skin. Lemon has clean, fresh, light, sharp top notes with slightly sweet, citrusy undertones. *S*

Neroli/Orange Blossom
(citrus bigardia/aurantium)

Traditionally used in wedding bouquets, neroli calms and soothes the skin. The delightful fragrance has delicate, fresh, floral top notes and warm, heady, bittersweet undertones.

Orange
(citrus sinensis)

This essential oil is distilled from the sweet orange variety. Orange shares some of the properties of neroli, and works well in skin toners and deodorants. It has sweet, fresh, fruity top notes and radiant, sensuous undertones.

Palmarosa
(cymbopogon martinii)

This is a delicate, gentle essential oil distilled from a grass closely related to lemongrass. Palmarosa has sweet, light, floral top notes with subtle lemon and geranium undertones.

Petitgrain
(citrus aurantium)

The refreshing aroma of petitgrain is often used in skin care products, and it has a relaxing, balancing quality. Petitgrain shares many of the qualities of neroli, and has fresh, floral, citrusy top notes and light, woody undertones.

Rose
(rosa centifolia/damascena)

Romantic rose has often been described as the queen of flowers, and it is best of all oils in skin care preparations. Rose has deep, sweet, floral top notes with dusky, honeyed undertones. *P*

Rosewood
(aniba rosaeodora)

Rosewood is an endangered species, so make sure the oil you buy comes from a sustainable rosewood plantation. Rosewood is both subtle and powerful with soft, floral top notes and sweet, woody undertones.

Sandalwood
(santalum album)

Sandalwood's warm, heavy fragrance increases over time, and it is beneficial for all skin types. Sandalwood has sweet, woody, roselike top notes and deep, balsamic, spicy, oriental undertones.

Ylang Ylang
(cananga odorata)

Ylang ylang is much used in the cosmetics industry for its voluptuous, exotic fragrance. It has intensely sweet, almond, floral, tropical top notes and slightly cloying, creamy, spicy undertones.

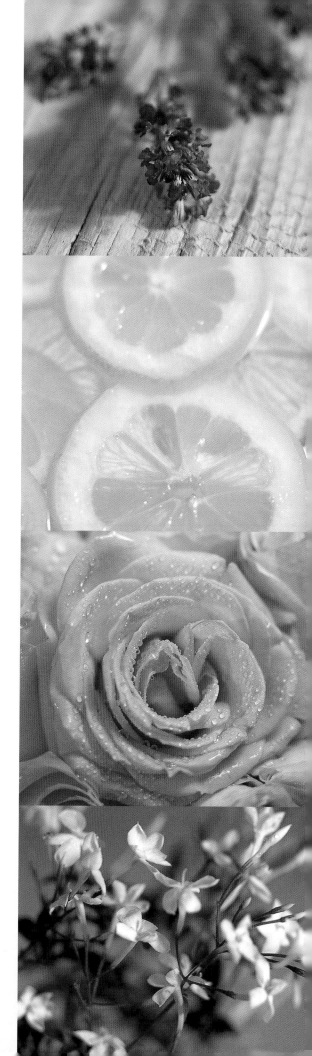

Equipment, Ingredients, and Containers

Equipment and Containers

Most of the equipment—and some of the ingredients—you need to make skin-care products can be found in the kitchen. A glass stirring rod is recommended, and can be purchased from one of the specialist suppliers listed on pages 124–125 or from a kitchen-supply store. You will also need to purchase a variety of glass jars in a range of different sizes, as these will be the containers for your skin creams, cleansers, and lip balms. Dark glass bottles, some with spray attachments and others with caps, are required for skin toners, body lotions, and deodorants.

Ingredients

All the ingredients below can be purchased from the specialist suppliers listed on pages 124–125, although some of these ingredients may also be found in your local natural-health store. Here are the main ingredients you will need to make your own cosmetics.

- Base products: skin lotion, cleanser, and cream, and hair shampoo and conditioner

- A range of essential oils, herbal tinctures, and flower waters

- Base oils: almond, apricot, rosehip seed, kukui nut, calendula, carrot, vitamin E, evening primrose, jojoba, avocado

- Beeswax, shea butter, Monoi de Tahiti, and cocoa butter

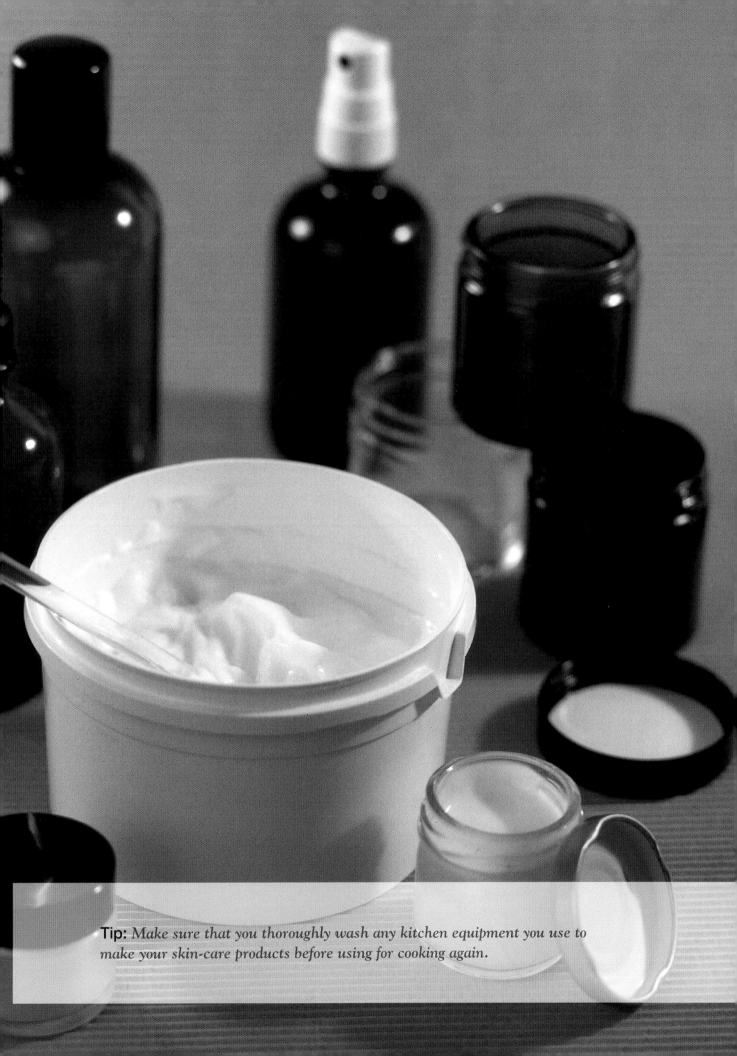

Tip: *Make sure that you thoroughly wash any kitchen equipment you use to make your skin-care products before using for cooking again.*

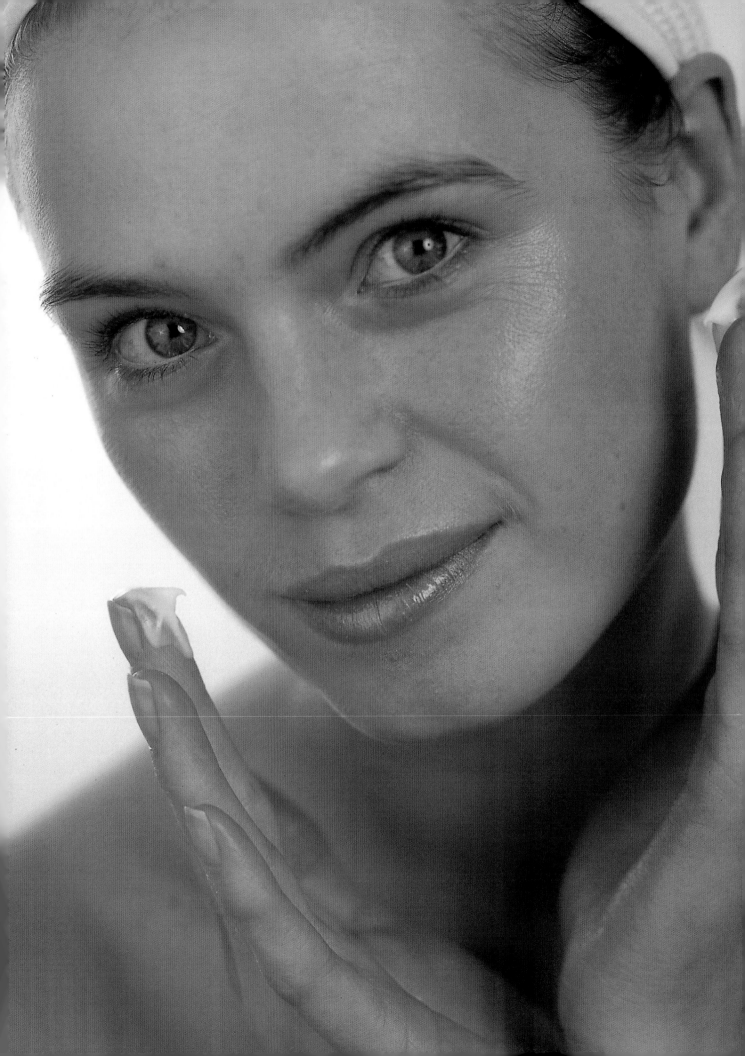

Chapter Two

Quick and Easy Daily Face Products

"The beauty of base products derives from simplicity; they are especially mild, gentle, and pure, making them great to use."

—Baldwins catalog

Creating Your Own Skin Care Cosmetics

The recipes in this chapter are quick and simple to make, so you can easily get started creating your own cosmetics. These recipes also provide a selection of daily cleansing, toning, and moisturizing products. They offer ideas for different additions to the base cleansers, toners, and moisturizers, so you can personalize all your face care products to suit your skin. By following a few easy, step-by-step instructions you can transform your daily face care regime.

You probably already know your skin type, and therefore which face care products are suitable for your face. However, it is a good idea to check the condition of your skin. Seasonal factors, such as turning on the central heating or spending time in the sun, affect the skin. Differences in temperature, whether the climate is damp or dry, and how much wind you are exposed to all affect the condition of your skin and especially your face. Therefore, several different kinds of cleansers, toners, and moisturizers can all have their uses at different times throughout the year.

You should also consider other factors that affect your skin, such as whether your general health is good and what types of food you eat. Taking a holistic approach to caring for your skin helps ensure you face the world looking as good as possible. This means looking at what you eat and making changes to help your skin from within. Some people can eat cream cakes and chips and still have a beautiful figure and lovely skin, but

they are in a tiny minority. Most of us need to eat sensibly to keep our bodies and our skin in good condition.

Alongside making your own daily face care products, you can make a few dietary changes. It is important to drink a lot of spring water. This flushes toxins out of the body through the urinary system, which means they don't have to be expelled through the skin. Reducing salt and caffeine and drinking herbal tea also helps. Eating less fried and processed foods, sugar, and red meat while increasing your consumption of organic fresh fruit and vegetables and whole grains can help bring a healthy glow to your face.

Another lifestyle factor that affects the skin is exercise. If you work in an office, the chances are you spend little time outside. Taking a daily walk in the park and escaping to the countryside is beneficial. This reduces exposure to air pollution and increases your intake of fresh air. Exercise generally stimulates the circulation and increases blood flow, which sends nutrients through the blood to nourish all parts of the body.

Making and using your own quick and easy daily face products, together with a few lifestyle changes, can improve the appearance of your face within a couple of weeks—all without expending too much time and effort. Caring for your face in this holistic way not only makes you look good but helps you feel healthy too.

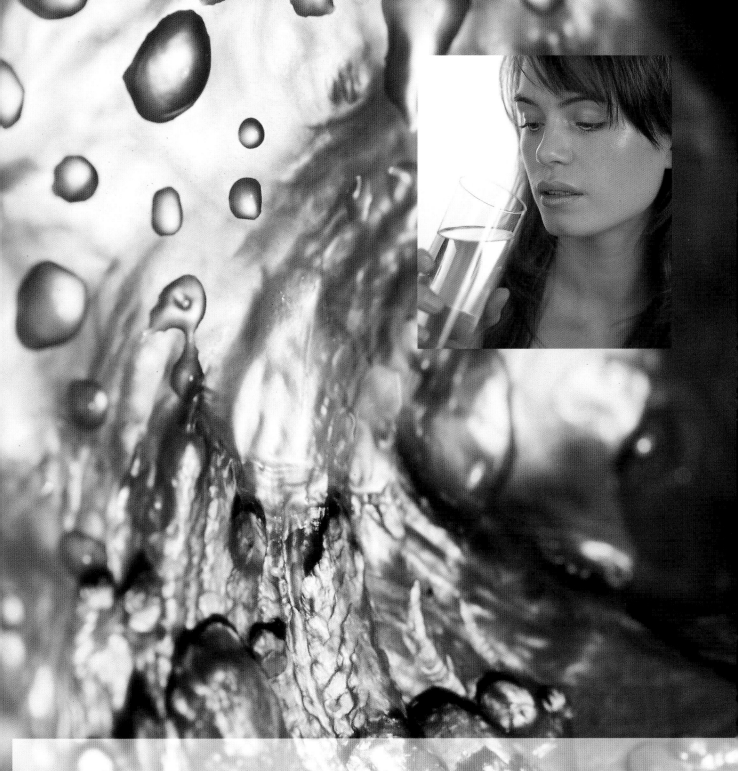

Tip: *As we age, our skin subtly changes without us really noticing. You need to take this into account by checking the condition of your skin before choosing your skin-care products and being prepared to modify your choice accordingly.*

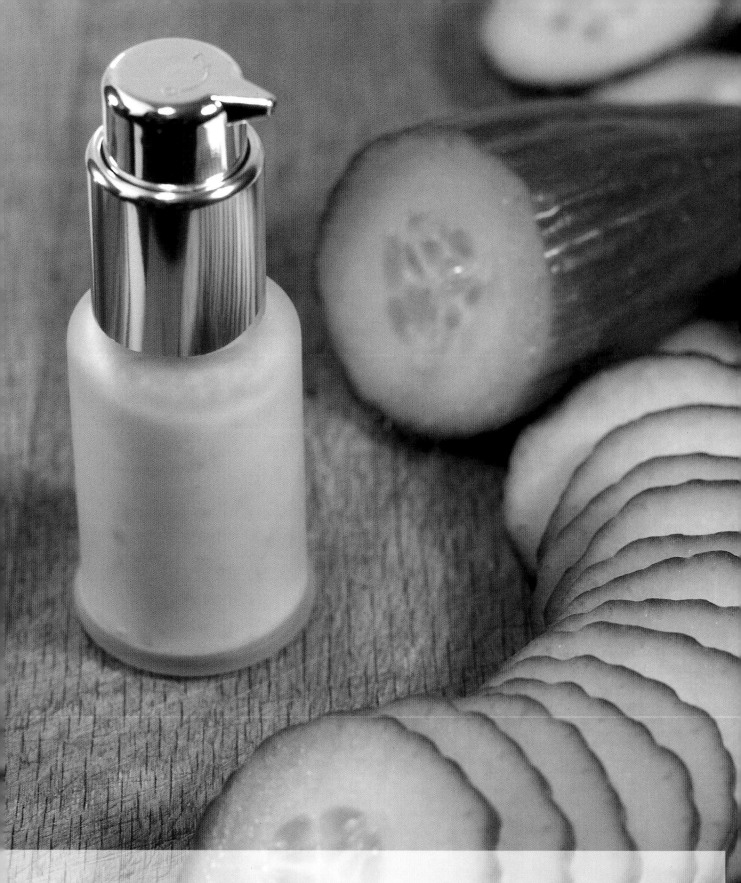

Tip: *To keep the cucumber and elderflower cleanser as fresh as possible, divide the amount you make into two portions. Pour one part into a bottle for current use and pour the other portion into another bottle that you can keep in the refrigerator until you are ready to use it.*

Face Cleansers

Cleansing the skin properly, especially the face, is fundamental to good skin care. This is even more important if you live in a city or near an industrial area, as airborne toxins will readily adhere to your face, causing damage and premature aging.

Cleansing is the first of the three step, twice daily face care regime of cleansing, toning, and moisturizing. Because facial skin is so delicate, soap is much too harsh and drying to use to wash the face.

Special face cleansers, mostly based around a cream or a lotion, are the best way to cleanse your face thoroughly yet gently. The following cleansers use a cleansing lotion base, and are best applied and wiped off with damp cotton balls.

Creamy Cucumber and Elderflower

Cucumber features in many commercial face cleansers, as it is a tried and trusted natural astringent and cleansing agent. Here, we use organic cucumber to create a fresh, natural cleanser, suitable for all skin types. Elderflowers are healing and astringent.

what's in it?
5 oz (150 ml) cleansing lotion base

⅓ of a fresh, organic cucumber

7 drops elderflower tincture

5 drops lemon essential oil

how's it made?
1 Wash the cucumber thoroughly in cold water. Chop a third of the cucumber roughly, place it in a blender, and puree.

2 Strain the cucumber through a piece of clean muslin. Squeeze the cloth to extract the juice.

3 Measure the cleansing lotion base into a glass container with a good pouring spout. Add the cucumber juice and stir thoroughly. Add the elderflower tincture and lemon oil and stir to thoroughly combine all the ingredients.

4 Pour the mixture into two bottles. Label them clearly. One is ready for use and the other can be stored in the refrigerator for up to one month.

Palmarosa and Linden Blossom

The fresh, clean smell of palmarosa blends beautifully with the sweet, slightly honeyed tones of linden flower water to create a delicate, fragrant cleanser, suitable for all skin types. Palmarosa is astringent, helps balance sebum production, and is reputed to help smooth out wrinkles.

what's in it?

5 oz (150 ml) cleansing lotion base

1 tbsp (15 ml) linden flower water

30 drops palmarosa

how's it made?

1 Measure the cleansing lotion base into a glass container with a good pouring spout.

2 Add the linden flower water and mix thoroughly. This will create a lotion rather than a cream. You could add a little less or a little more flower water according to preference.

3 Add the drops of palmarosa carefully, and stir well to incorporate thoroughly into the mixture.

4 Pour into a bottle and label. The cleanser is ready to use.

Mild Meadowsweet

Meadowsweet is anti-inflammatory and astringent, and makes a useful addition to this cleanser. Meadowsweet is also mildly analgesic because it contains salicylic acid—nature's own natural aspirin. The addition of rose flower water and neroli make this gentle, sweet smelling cleanser especially mild and suited to sensitive, inflamed, or irritated skin.

what's in it?

5 oz (150 ml) cleansing lotion base

10 drops meadowsweet tincture

1 tbsp (15 ml) rose flower water

20 drops neroli

how's it made?

1 Measure the cleansing lotion base into a glass container with a good pouring spout.

2 Add the rose flower water and mix thoroughly. This will create a lotion rather than a cream. You could add a little less or a little more flower water according to preference.

3 Add the drops of neroli and meadowsweet carefully, and stir well to incorporate thoroughly into the mixture.

4 Pour into a bottle and label. The cleanser is ready to use.

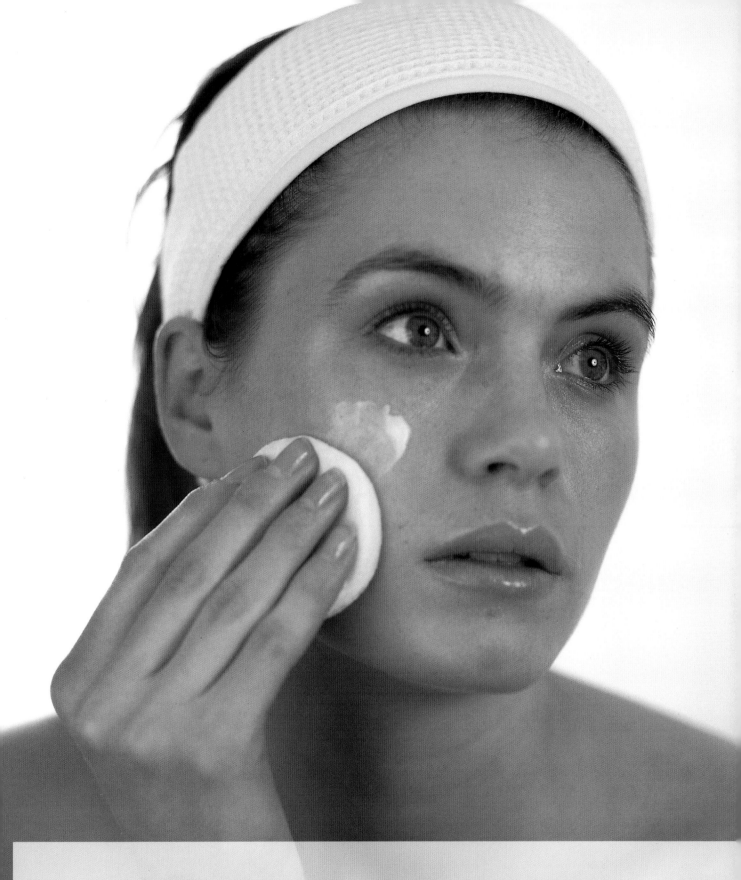

Did You Know? *Palmarosa is one of a few essential oils that helps keep the skin clear and fresh by stimulating healthy cellular regeneration.*

Tip: *Eyebright also helps eyes that have a tendency for weepiness caused by sensitivity to light, so this is a good eye cleanser if your eyes are light sensitive.*

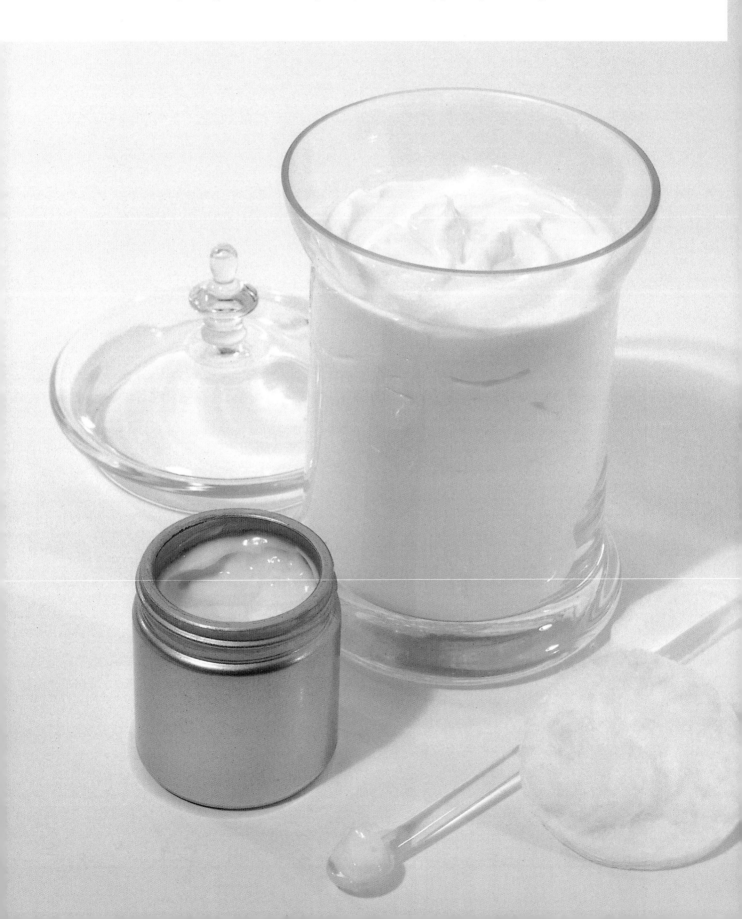

Eye Area Cleansers

The delicate skin around the eyes needs extra special care and attention. Some commercial cleansers contain harsh ingredients or a high percentage of alcohol, which are quite unsuitable for the delicate area around the eyes. The following two cleansers contain gentle oils, flower waters, and herbal tinctures that are especially suited to gently cleansing the eye area.

However, as with all face care products, care must be taken not to get any of the eye cleanser into the eyes themselves.

If you accidentally rub a little cleanser into your eyes, simply rinse out with cold water and pat the eyes dry. Use damp cotton balls to apply and wipe off the eye area cleansers.

Gentle Eyebright

As the name suggests, eyebright is a herb that has a special affinity with the eyes. It is especially helpful if there is any inflammation or stinging around the eyes. In this cleanser, tincture of eyebright is mixed with an infusion of chamomile to create a gentle cleanser suitable for the eye area, especially if the eyes are red and tired.

what's in it?
2 tbsp (25 ml) cleansing lotion base
2 drops eyebright tincture
1 tsp (5 ml) chamomile infusion (see step 3)

how's it made?
1 Measure the cleansing lotion base into a 2 oz (50 ml) glass jar.

2 Add the eyebright tincture to the base lotion. Mix thoroughly.

3 Make an infusion of chamomile by steeping one organic chamomile tea bag for ten minutes. Let cool and stir 1 tsp (5 ml) of the infusion thoroughly into the eye cleanser.

4 Pour the cleanser into a jar and label it. The eye area cleanser is ready to use.

Evening Primrose and Cornflower Water

Evening primrose oil is rich in gamma linoleic acid, an essential fatty acid. It has been shown to help psoriasis, eczema, and other skin conditions, and is generally useful for sensitive, delicate skin. The clean, fresh scent of cornflower water also lightly fragrances this eye area cleanser.

what's in it?

2 tbsp (25 ml) cleansing lotion base

1 evening primrose oil capsule

1 tsp (5 ml) cornflower water

how's it made?

1 Measure the cleansing lotion base into a 2 oz (50 ml) glass jar.

2 Pierce the capsule of evening primrose oil with a pin and squeeze out the oil into the base lotion. Mix thoroughly.

3 Add the cornflower water to the mixture and stir thoroughly.

4 Pour the cleanser into a jar and label it. The eye area cleanser is ready to use.

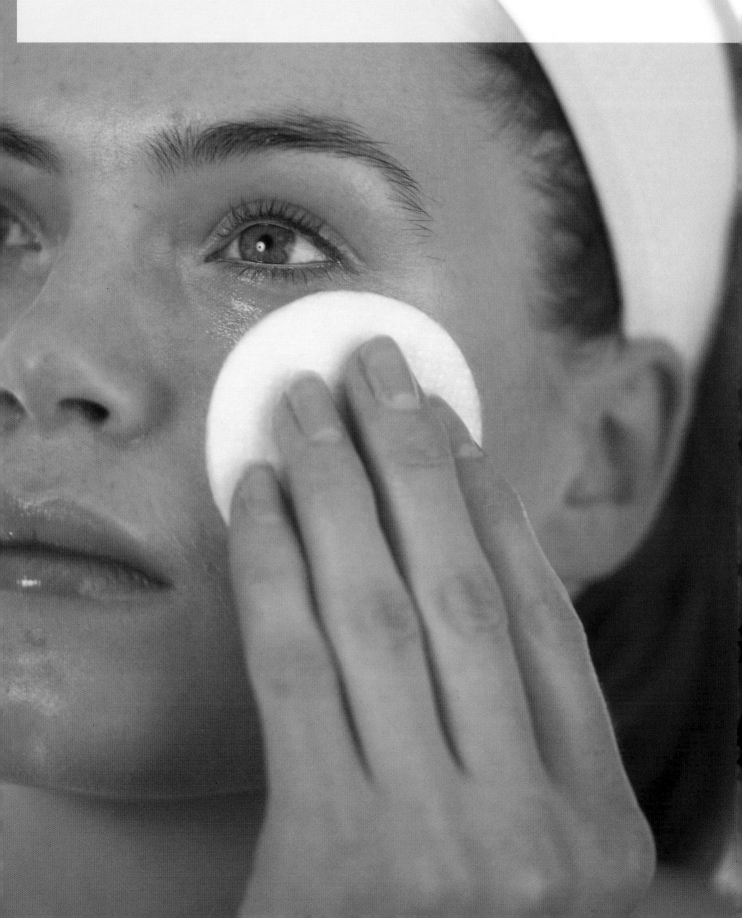

Tip: *Cornflower water has traditionally been used to soothe tired eyes, help eye infections, and provide general care for the eye area.*

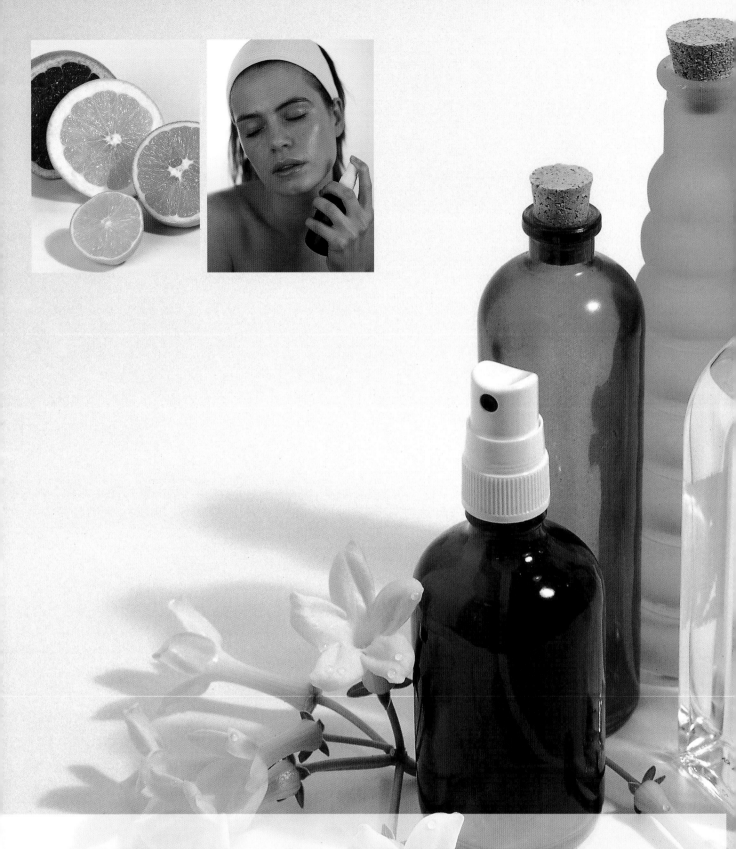

Did You Know? *Orange flower water is obtained by distillation of orange blossom petals. This distillation process is actually undertaken to produce the essential oil neroli. The orange flower water is considered a by-product of this process, although it is valuable in its own right. Using products containing both neroli and orange flower water utilizes the synergy of the whole plant.*

Toners

Skin toners are used to tighten the skin's pores after cleansing. Toners also function to remove traces of cleanser, so they are a valuable part of a skin care regime. However, many store-bought toners contain harsh ingredients that dry the skin, leaving your face feeling dry and tight.

Making your own skin toners is a simple process, and well worth the effort. By using some of the recipes that follow, you can be sure you are using only pure, natural, and organic ingredients that are kind and gentle to your skin and of benefit to your complexion.

Fresh and Fruity

This fresh smelling skin toner is a treat to use in the morning, as the fragrance is uplifting and invigorating. This astringent toner is ideal for youthful and oily skins, though it is gentle enough for all skin types. The addition of citrus essential oils helps tone the complexion, and leaves your skin feeling clean and refreshed.

what's in it?

1 tbsp (10 ml) high proof vodka

2 drops grapefruit

2 drops neroli

2 drops orange

2 drops lemon

2 tbsp (25 ml) witch hazel

1 cup (250 ml) orange flower water

how's it made?

1 Pour the high proof vodka into a clean, dry glass bottle large enough to hold at least 11 oz (300 ml) of liquid. You can use a spray bottle to easily apply the toner.

2 Add the essential oils to the vodka and shake vigorously to dissolve the oils.

3 Add the witch hazel and shake well, followed by the orange flower water. Shake the bottle until all the ingredients have blended together well.

4 The skin toner is ready to use. However, the essential oils will separate slightly over time, so shake the bottle just before using each time.

Rose and Geranium Toner

This skin toner is suited to all skin types, as the main action of the essential oils is balancing. However, rose is also especially suited to dry and mature skin. The deep, honeyed aroma of roses from both rose essential oil and from the rose water mingles with the fresh, floral scent of geranium to make a delightful, delicate skin toner.

what's in it?
1 tbsp (10 ml) high proof vodka

4 drops rose

4 drops geranium

2 tbsp (25 ml) witch hazel

1 cup (250 ml) rose flower water

how's it made?

1 Pour the high proof vodka into a clean, dry glass bottle large enough to hold at least 11 oz (300 ml) of liquid. You can use a spray bottle to easily apply the toner.

2 Add the essential oils to the vodka and shake vigorously to dissolve the oils.

3 Add the witch hazel and shake well, followed by the rose flower water. Shake the bottle until all the ingredients have blended together well.

4 The skin toner is ready to use. However, the essential oils will separate slightly over time, so shake the bottle just before using each time.

Orange Flower Blossom and Petitgrain

The fresh, woody smell of petitgrain in this skin toner is complemented by the sweet, delicate scent of neroli. The gentle action of linden flower water makes this toner suitable for all skin types, but it is especially great for dry and sensitive skin. The sweet, honeyed fragrance of linden blossom blends with palmarosa and chamomile to give a balanced overall fragrance.

what's in it?
1 tbsp (10 ml) high proof vodka

2 drops neroli

2 drops petitgrain

2 drops chamomile

2 drops palmarosa

2 tbsp (25 ml) witch hazel

1 cup (250 ml) linden flower water

how's it made?

1 Pour the high proof vodka into a clean, dry glass bottle large enough to hold at least 11 oz (300 ml) of liquid. You can use a spray bottle to easily apply the toner.

2 Add the essential oils to the vodka and shake vigorously to dissolve the oils.

3 Add the witch hazel and shake well, followed by the linden flower water. Shake the bottle until all the ingredients have blended together well.

4 The skin toner is ready to use. However, the essential oils will separate slightly over time, so shake the bottle just before using each time.

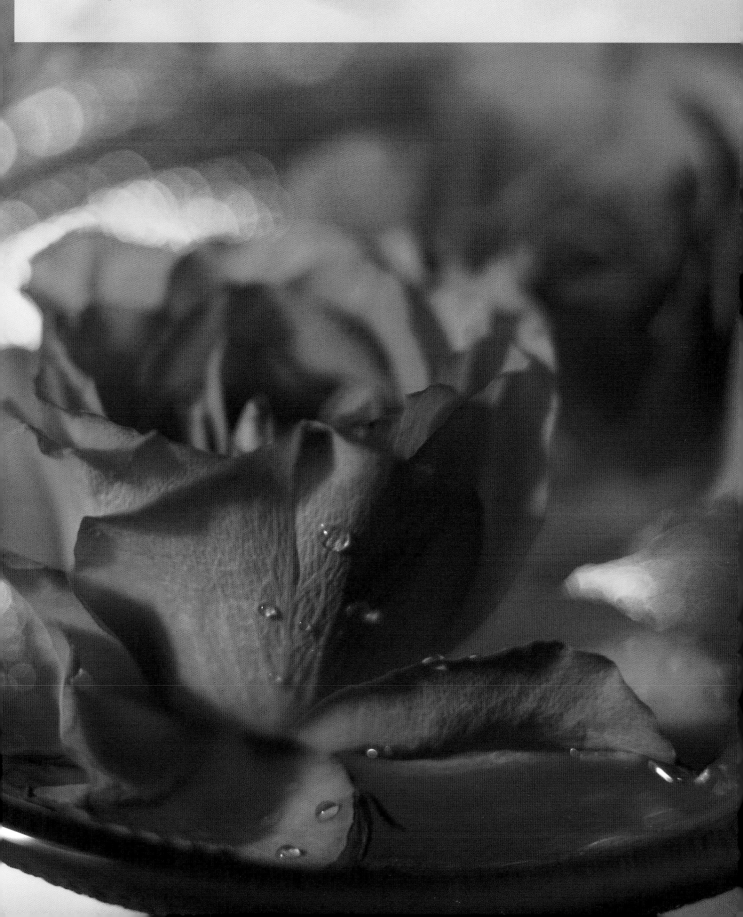

Did You Know? *Skin toners are wonderfully cooling and refreshing when sprayed on the face on a hot, sunny day.*

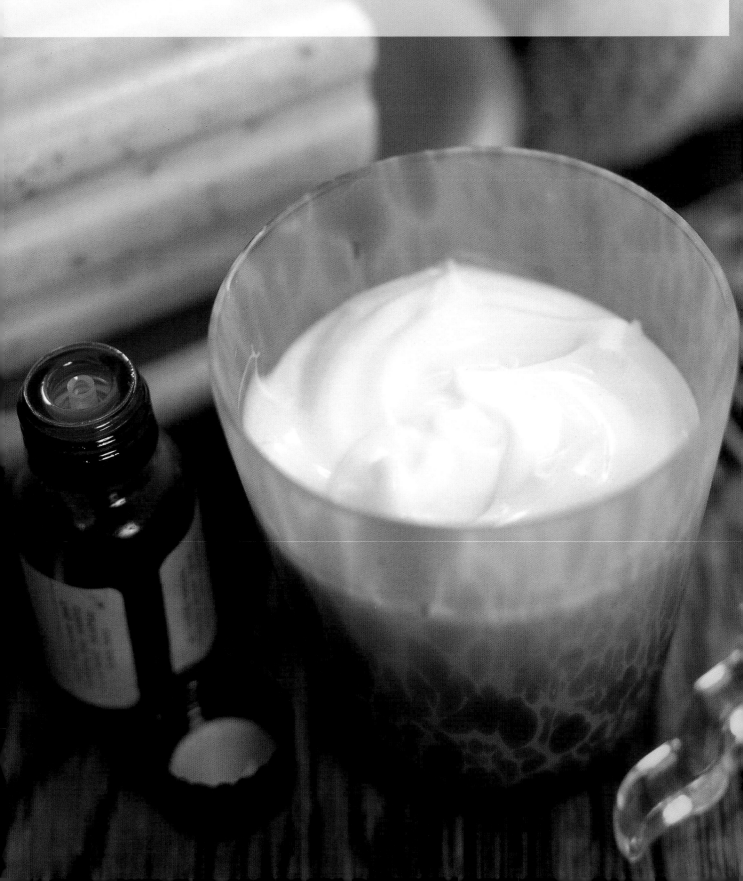

Did You Know? *The extensive reputation of sandalwood as a perfume is partly due to its fragrance, which appeals to both women and men. However, sandalwood's sweet, woody perfume is reputed to be an aphrodisiac, and its popularity is perhaps a testament to this quality.*

Moisturizing Creams

In many ways, moisturizers are the most impor-tant product throughout the whole skin-care range. They nourish, hydrate, and protect the skin, and keep it supple and able to fulfill its functions for the body.

If you were stuck on a desert island and could take only one skin-care product with you, it would have to be a good, basic moisturizer.

The moisturizer recipes here are really quick and simple to make. Before starting, you need to buy a cream base from a reputable supplier (see pages 124–125). Most suppliers offer at least two cream bases—a light one and a richer, heavier one. This will give you a lighter day moisturizer and a richer night cream. Choose the cream that suits your skin best, or make up different moisturizers by combining both types.

Kukui Nut and Sandalwood

Kukui nut oil is high in linoleic and linolenic fatty acids, which are essential for healthy skin. Kukui nut oil is also easily absorbed by the skin and is known to benefit acne, eczema, and pso-riasis. Sandalwood is much used in skin care and is beneficial for all skin types, especially helping oily skin as it is slightly astringent. This cream is suited to all skin types and both sexes, so it makes a good general moisturizer for every-one in the family.

what's in it?
2 tbsp (30 gm) of your chosen cream base

1 tsp (2 ml) kukui nut oil

12 drops sandalwood

how's it made?

1 Half fill a clean glass jar (either a 2 or 2½ oz [50 or 60 gm] size) with your chosen cream base.

2 Stir in the kukui nut oil using a glass stirring rod or a chopstick. Make sure the oil is thor-oughly blended into the cream.

3 Carefully add the sandalwood. Stir in thor-oughly, making sure the essential oil is com-pletely dispersed throughout the cream. The cream is now ready to use.

Calendula and Neroli

The addition of macerated calendula oil gives this cream healing and anti-inflammatory properties, and it soothes and softens the skin. Neroli essential oil gives a delicate, sweet scent. Neroli is calming and good for nerves, and it soothes sensitive, delicate skin. Neroli also helps in the regeneration of new skin cells, which keeps the skin looking fresh and smooth. This moisturizer is particularly suited to dry, sensitive skin, and for sore or chapped skin, redness, or broken thread veins.

what's in it?
2 tbsp (30 gm) of your chosen cream base

1 tsp (3 ml) macerated calendula oil

10 drops neroli

how's it made?

1 Half fill a clean glass jar (either a 2 or 2½ oz [50 or 60 gm] size) with your chosen cream base.

2 Stir in the calendula oil using a glass stirring rod or a chopstick. Make sure the oil is thoroughly blended into the cream.

3 Carefully add the neroli. Stir in thoroughly, making sure the essential oil is thoroughly dispersed throughout the cream. The cream is ready to use.

Rosewood and Rose with Rosehip Seed Oil

The wonderful fragrance of rose is balanced with the woody, floral perfume of rosewood. Together they produce a delicate feminine perfume. Both these oils are excellent in face creams. Rosehip seed oil is rich in G.L.A. or gamma linoleic acid, which is valuable in treating a variety of skin problems, especially if there is inflammation. This cream is particularly suited to dry, sensitive, or mature skin, but makes a beautiful moisturizer for all skin types.

what's in it?
2 tbsp (30 gm) of your chosen cream base

1 tsp (3 ml) rosehip seed oil

4 drops rose

7 drops rosewood

how's it made?

1 Half fill a clean glass jar (either a 2 or 2½ oz [50 or 60 gm] size) with your chosen cream base.

2 Stir in the rosehip seed oil using a glass stirring rod or a chopstick. Make sure the oil is thoroughly blended into the cream.

3 Carefully add the rose and rosewood. Stir in thoroughly, making sure the essential oils are completely dispersed throughout the cream. The cream is ready to use.

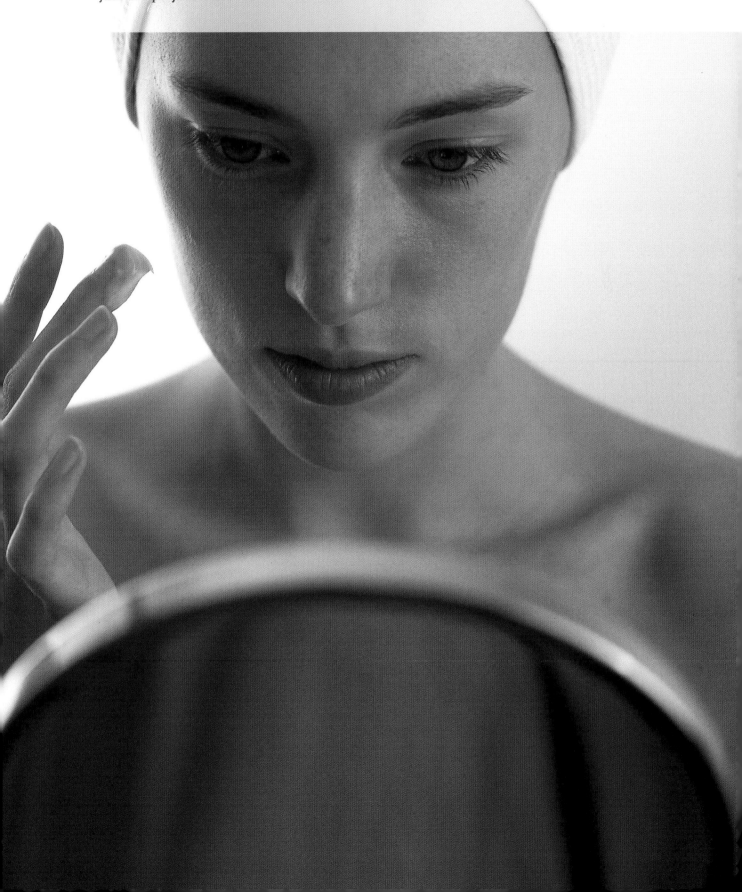

Did You Know? *Neroli is distilled from the flowers of the bitter orange, which has grown for centuries around Seville. This hauntingly beautiful fragranced essential oil is named after an Italian princess who used it as her favorite perfume.*

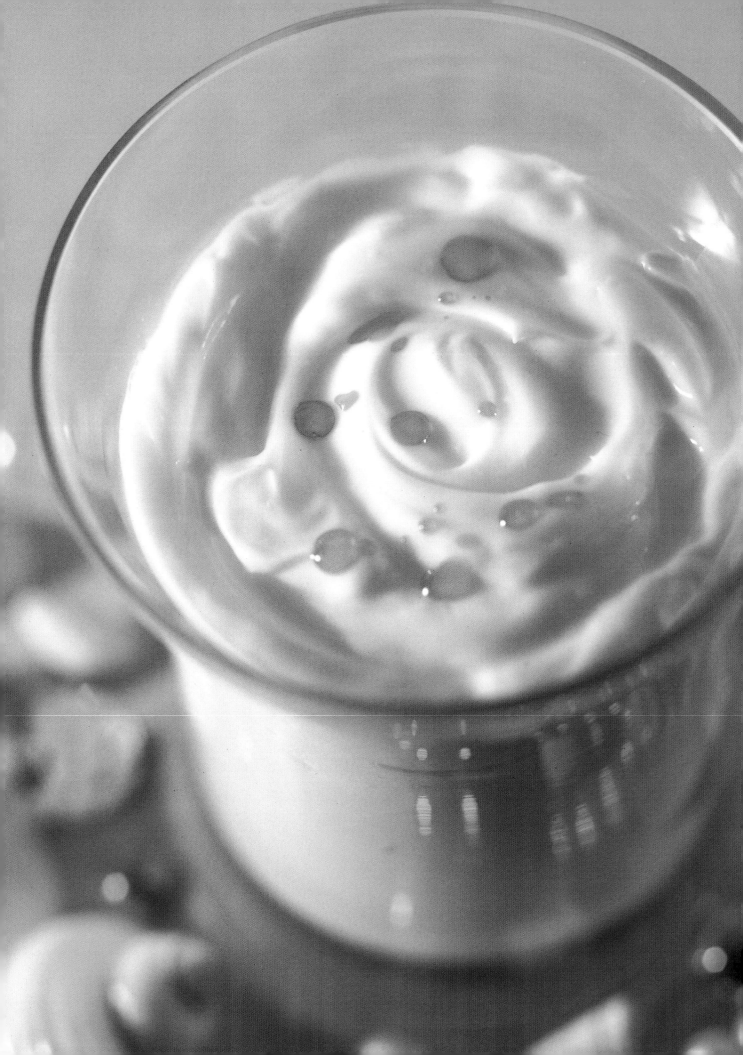

Chapter Three

Making Creams, Lotions, and Lip Balms

"Since essential oils are soluble in oil and alcohol and impart their scent to water, they provide the ideal ingredient for cosmetics and general skin care."

–Julia Lawless, *author and aromatherapist*

Homemade Face Creams

Making your own skin-care products can be very rewarding. Although it is fun to experiment with the wide range of commercial skin-care creams and lotions available these days, they are often expensive. In addition, you are probably not familiar with some of the ingredients the creams are made from, and many of these substances are inorganic and synthetic. If you develop a skin rash or allergy from using a store-bought cream, not only do you not know exactly what caused it but you have to throw away what was probably an expensive item.

Creating you own creams, lotions, and balms from scratch means you have the satisfaction of knowing every single ingredient that has gone into the making of the product. You can ensure that you use only pure, natural, plant-based constituents, and you can choose organic ingredients whenever possible. The chances of developing an allergic reaction to your own homemade face creams and body lotions are far less than if you use many of the store-bought skin-care products.

Incorporating essential oils for their skin-care properties enriches the creams and lotions, provides natural healing qualities, and imparts a natural fragrance. The wide range of essential oils available gives you the flexibility to make a variety of skin-care products for different skin types from a few basic formulas. In this way, you end up with high-quality, natural skin creams and lotions at a much cheaper cost than their commercial equivalents.

However, there is one minor drawback in making your own face creams. Commercial face-cream manufacturers use specialized equipment, including emulsifying machines. These help the fat-based ingredients and the water-based ingredients blend into the light, fluffy, homogenous face creams you usually purchase. Your homemade creams will not emulsify in quite the same way.

This means you will end up with quite oily creams in some instances, as not all the fat-based ingredients will emulsify fully with the water-based ingredients. This doesn't make the cream any less effective, but it does take longer for it to absorb into the skin. This can be ideal; for example gardeners or manual workers, who often have very dry, cracked skin, will enjoy the hand creams as their skin will readily absorb these rich creams.

The best thing to do is to experiment. If you find any of your homemade face or hand creams too rich, or they take too long to absorb into your skin, mix them into a cream base. Try half and half to start with, and adjust the proportion of cream base to homemade cream to get exactly the texture that suits your skin best. With a bit of experimentation, you will end up with a selection of natural, beautifully fragranced skin creams that suit your own individual skin type and condition.

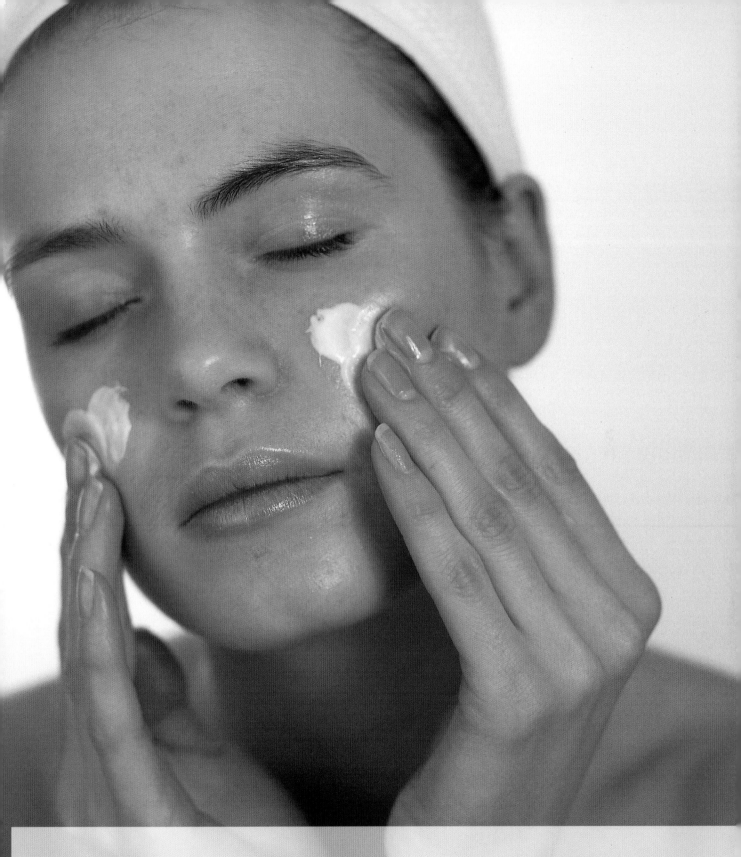

Tip: *In some recipes, liquids are measured by volume and in others they are measured by weight. This makes no difference to the creams; it's simply how the different recipes were originally formulated.*

Tip: *Jojoba oil contains approximately four times the amount of waxy esters contained within the skin's sebum. Incorporating jojoba oil into skin creams not only protects the skin but allows the skin a chance to heal and repair itself.*

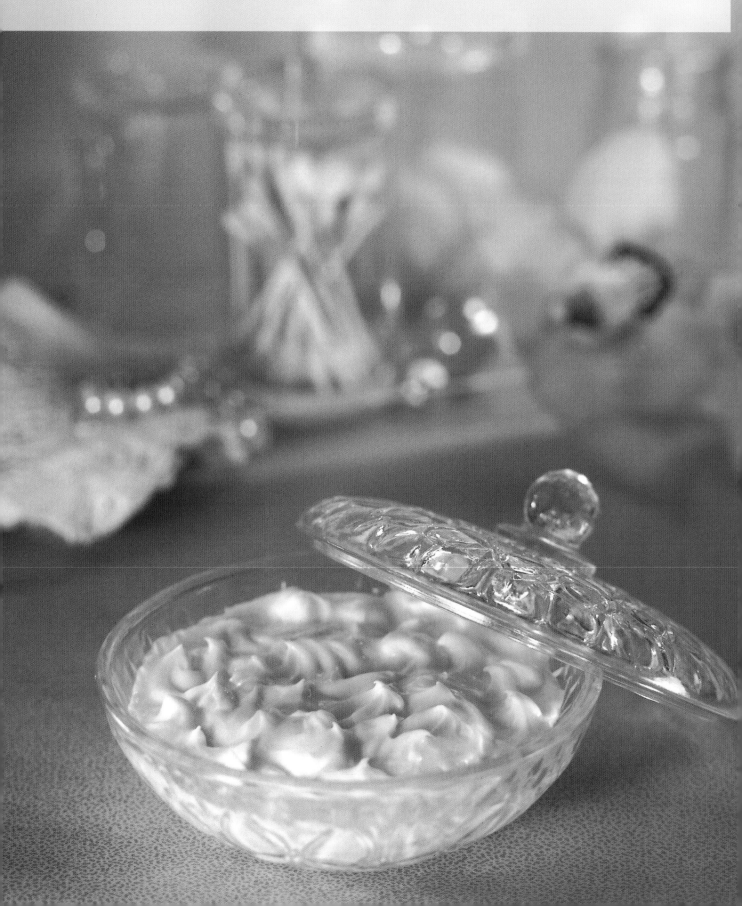

Creams

Face creams fall into two main types: moisturizers and cleansers. Although there are commercially available face cleansers that are clear, noncreamy liquids, these are often alcohol based. They effectively clean the face, but leave the skin dry and stripped of naturally occurring sebum. These are marketed at those with oily skin, or with acne, as they are supposed to reduce oiliness, but they only provide a temporary solution and are too harsh for the skin. Cream-based cleansers are much kinder to the skin and they are equally effective at cleansing deep into the pores.

All moisturizing products are cream based. The process involves warming the fat-based ingredients—such as cocoa butter and almond oil—and the water-based ingredients—such as rose water or orange flower water—separately. These are then mixed together by dripping the latter slowly into the former, beating the mixture continuously.

Cocoa Butter and Rose Cream

This is a rich face cream that is especially suited to dry and mature skin. At the end of winter, when the face has been exposed to the drying effects of cold wind, rain, and central heating, the skin may be very dry and perhaps a little red or flaky. This lovely recipe contains both essential and base oils that have a gentle, deep, and lasting action on the skin, making the cream a really effective moisturizer.

what's in it?

1 tsp (4 gm) yellow beeswax	2 tbsp (35 ml) almond oil
½ cup (130 ml) rose water	1 tbsp (10 ml) jojoba oil
1 tbsp (10 ml) glycerin	15 drops rose
1½ tbsp (20 gm) cocoa butter	15 drops frankincense
	5 drops chamomile

how's it made?

1 Melt the beeswax in a bowl placed in a baking tray of hot water over a gentle heat.

2 Heat the rose water and glycerin in another bowl alongside the melting beeswax.

3 Once the beeswax has melted, add the cocoa butter, stirring constantly until it is melted. Then add the almond and jojoba oils, beating the mixture steadily to ensure all ingredients are thoroughly incorporated.

4 Once the contents of both bowls are the same temperature (warmed through but not simmering) add the rose water and glycerin, drop by drop, into the oils. Beat steadily. An assistant can be useful at this stage, or you can even use an electric beater if you have one with a very low setting.

5 When all the rose water and glycerin have been beaten into the oils, remove from the heat, stirring until the mixture has cooled. Then add the essential oils, mixing them in thoroughly, and then pour into glass jars. Put the lids on once the cream is quite cool, label the jars, and the cream is ready to use.

Neroli and Petitgrain Cream Cleanser

This cleanser incorporates the nourishing oils of avocado and wheatgerm. Avocado oil regenerates skin cells and has skin softening and healing qualities. It is rich in vitamins A, D, and E, which are all beneficial for healthy skin. Wheatgerm oil contains carotene and vegetable lecithin, which help prevent moisture loss from the skin. The fragrance is delicate and floral.

what's in it?

½ oz (18 gm) yellow beeswax

1 tbsp (60 ml) orange flower water

4 tbsp (60 ml) avocado oil

2 tbsp (30 ml) wheatgerm oil

5 drops neroli

6 drops petitgrain

how's it made?

1 Melt the beeswax in a bowl placed in a baking tray of hot water over a gentle heat.

2 Heat the orange flower water in another small bowl alongside the melting beeswax.

3 Once the beeswax has melted, add the avocado and wheatgerm oils, beating the mixture to ensure the ingredients are thoroughly blended.

4 Once the contents of both bowls are the same temperature (warmed through but not simmering) add the orange flower water, drop by drop, into the oils. Beat steadily. An assistant can be useful at this stage, or you can even use an electric beater if you have one with a very low setting.

5 When all the flower water has been beaten into the oils, remove from the heat, stirring until the mixture has cooled. Then add the essential oils, mixing them in thoroughly, and then pour into glass jars. Put the lids on once the cream is quite cool, label the jars, and the cream is ready to use.

Almond Oil and Rosehip Seed Cream

The oil extracted from the Rosa Mosquetta rosehip seed is much valued for its skin-regeneration properties. Here, it is combined with almond oil to make a nourishing face cream suitable for all skin types. Delicate neroli is blended with lavender and a hint of ylang ylang to create a finely perfumed cream.

what's in it?

1½ tsp (5 gm) yellow beeswax

1 tbsp (15 gm) rose water

2 tbsp (30 gm) almond oil

2 tsp (10 gm) rosehip seed oil, preferably Rosa Mosquetta

2 vitamin E capsules

10 drops neroli

10 drops lavender

5 drops ylang ylang

how's it made?

1 Melt the beeswax in a bowl placed in a baking tray of hot water over a gentle heat.

2 Heat the rose water in another bowl alongside the melting beeswax.

3 Once the beeswax has melted, add the almond and rosehip seed oils, beating the mixture steadily to ensure they are incorporated thoroughly. Prick open the vitamin E capsules with a pin and squeeze into the mixture.

4 Once the contents of both bowls are the same temperature (warmed through but simmering) add the rose water, drop by drop, into the oils. Beat steadily. An assistant can be useful at this stage, or you can even use an electric beater if you have one with a very low setting.

5 When all the flower water has been beaten into the oils, remove from the heat, stirring until the mixture has cooled. Then add the essential oils, mixing them in thoroughly, and then pour into glass jars. Put the lids on once the cream is quite cool, label the jars, and the cream is ready to use.

Did You Know? *Wheatgerm oil is a natural antioxidant and it helps preserve the shelf life of the cream.*

Did You Know? *Honey is a natural moisturizer that hydrates and soothes the skin. It also inhibits the growth of bacteria.*

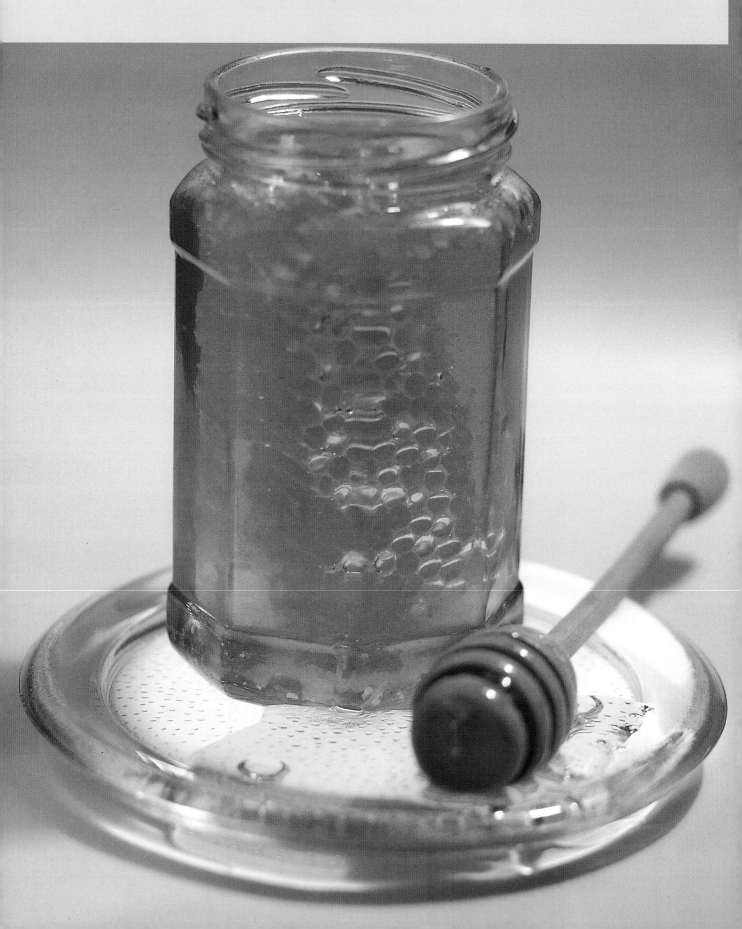

Shea Butter and Honey Antiwrinkle Cream

The healing properties of shea butter, or karite butter, have been used in skin care for centuries in central Africa. Shea butter has a gentle but effective moisturizing action, and is suitable for sensitive and dry skin that is prone to wrinkles. Combined with the healing properties of honey, this cream is a valuable cosmetic you will come to rely on to soften and soothe your skin.

what's in it?

2 tsp (7 gm) yellow beeswax	3 tsp (15 ml) almond oil
3 tsp (15 ml) linden flower water	2 tsp (10 ml) wheatgerm oil
1 tsp (5 ml) warmed liquid honey	2 drops myrrh
3 tsp (15 gm) shea butter	3 drops jasmine

how's it made?

1 Melt the beeswax in a bowl placed in a baking tray of hot water over a gentle heat.

2 Heat the linden flower water and honey in another bowl alongside the melting beeswax.

3 Once the beeswax has melted, add the shea butter, stirring constantly until it is melted. Then add the almond and wheatgerm oils, beating the mixture steadily to ensure all ingredients are thoroughly incorporated.

4 Once the contents of both bowls are the same temperature (warmed through but not simmering) add the linden flower water and honey, drop by drop, into the oils. Beat steadily. An assistant can be useful at this stage, or you can even use an electric beater if you have one with a very low setting.

5 When all the linden flower water and honey have been beaten into the oils, remove from the heat, stirring until the mixture has cooled. Then add the essential oils, mixing them in thoroughly, and then pour into glass jars. Put the lids on once the cream is quite cool, label the jars, and the cream is ready to use.

Galen's Cold Cream

This recipe is based on the original Galen's Cold Cream, which is thousands of years old. The cream sets firm but liquefies on contact with the natural warmth of the skin. Galen's Cold Cream is a good cleansing cream for mature and dry skin. Rose oil gives a wonderful and luxurious fragrance, making this cleanser a real treat to use.

what's in it?

2 tsp (10 gm) yellow beeswax
2 tbsp (30 gm) rose water
3 tbsp (40 gm) almond oil
10 drops rose

how's it made?

1 Melt the beeswax in a bowl placed in a baking tray of hot water over a gentle heat.

2 Heat the rose water in a second small bowl alongside the bowl of melting beeswax.

3 Once the beeswax has melted, add the almond oil, beating the mixture steadily to ensure the ingredients are thoroughly incorporated.

4 Once the contents of both bowls are the same temperature (warmed through but not simmering) add the rose water, drop by drop, into the oil. Beat steadily. An assistant can be useful at this stage, or you can use an electric beater if you have one with a very low setting.

5 When all the rose water has been beaten into the oil, remove from the heat, stirring until the mixture has cooled. Then add the rose, mixing it in thoroughly, and then pour into glass jars. Put the lids on once the cream is quite cool, label the jars, and the cream is ready to use.

Coconut Oil Hand Cream

This is a very simple cream to make as there is no flower water or beeswax to incorporate. The cream sets easily because coconut oil is solid at room temperature, but the cream easily liquefies on contact with the warmth of the skin. Lemon oil is fresh smelling and gently helps fade any discolored skin on the hands. It blends into a refreshing floral fragrance with the lavender.

what's in it?

5 tbsp (75 gm) coconut oil

1½ tbsp (25 gm) almond oil

10 drops lemon

10 drops lavender

how's it made?

1 Use a double boiler if you have one, or put a small saucepan inside a larger saucepan that is half filled with hot water. Add the coconut oil to the small saucepan and warm gently over a low heat until the coconut oil has melted.

2 Slowly pour in the almond oil, mixing continuously until the mixture is blended.

3 Remove from the heat and stir in the essential oils, mixing them in thoroughly, and pour into glass jars.

4 Put the lids on once the cream is quite cool, label the jars, and the cream is ready to use.

Geranium and Myrrh Hand Cream

This is another easy cream to make. It is excellent for those who work outdoors with their hands. The skin on the hands can easily become hard, dry, and chapped or cracked if it is not cared for properly. This hand cream is deeply penetrating and moisturizing, and the myrrh helps heal any small cuts, cracks, or lesions on the skin.

what's in it?

2 tsp (10 gm) yellow beeswax

4 tbsp (50 gm) cocoa butter

3 tbsp (40 ml) almond oil

1 tsp (5 ml) infused calendula oil

1 tsp (5 ml) glycerin

10 drops myrrh

10 drops geranium

how's it made?

1 Melt the beeswax in a bowl placed in a baking tray of hot water over a gentle heat.

2 Once the beeswax has melted, add the cocoa butter, stirring constantly until it is melted. Then add the almond oil and calendula oil, beating the mixture steadily to ensure all ingredients are thoroughly incorporated.

3 Add the glycerin to the oils in a slow trickle, beating steadily.

4 Once all the glycerin has been beaten into the oils, remove from the heat, stirring until the mixture has cooled. Then add the essential oils, mixing them in thoroughly, and then pour into glass jars. Put the lids on once the cream is quite cool, label the jars, and the cream is ready to use.

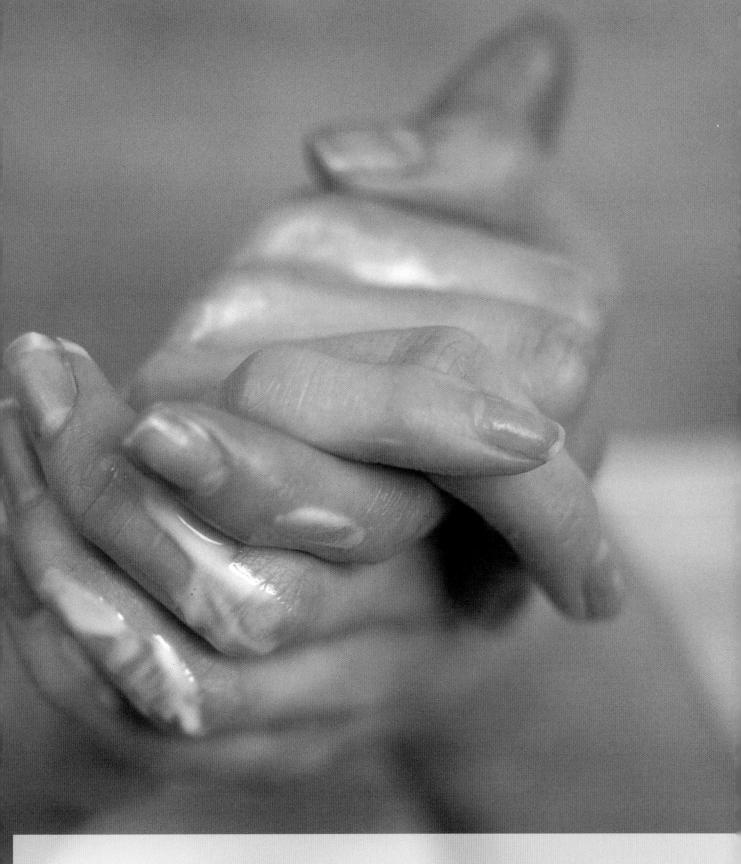

Tip: *Coconut Oil Hand Cream is also very good for the feet. After scrubbing away the hard, dead skin on the soles of the feet, apply the coconut oil cream for a deeply moisturizing treatment.*

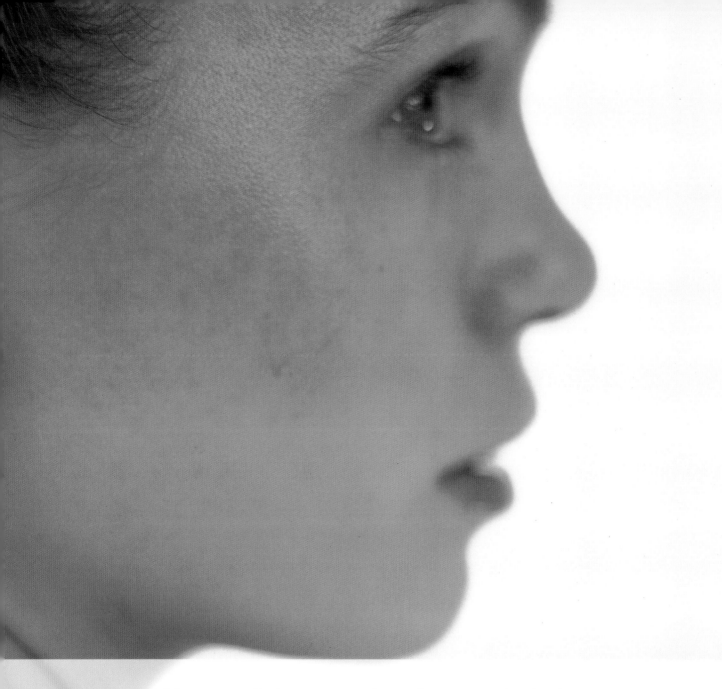

Tip: *Make sure you don't expose your skin to the sun immediately after using the lotion on page 55. It contains bergamot, a photosensitizer that could cause skin discoloration if used on the skin in strong sunlight.*

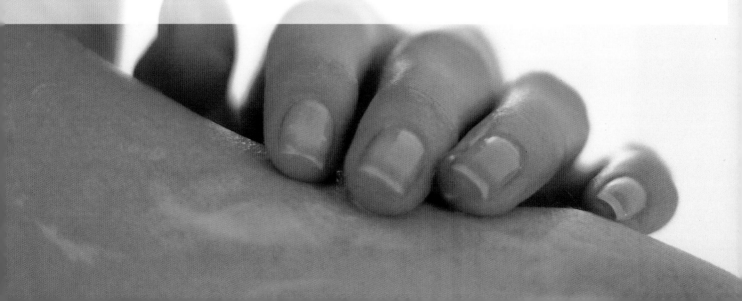

Lotions

Body lotions are moisturizers for the body. Lotions are thinner than face creams, so they spread easily over the larger areas of the body. Easy to apply, they are absorbed quickly by the skin. Body lotions are valuable in the summer when the sun has dried the skin, especially if you have been sunbathing. The body does need moisturizing all year round however, and body lotions provide a good way to moisturize the skin.

The following recipes can be made by using either a lotion base or thinning one of your homemade face or hand creams with flower water. Lotion base is ready to be used immediately in the recipes, and is quick and simple to use. If you would like to use one of your homemade creams, put a suitable quantity into a small glass jar. Put this in a container of hot water until the cream has softened or melted. Then beat in a flower water of your choice until you have the desired thickness of lotion. Use only half the quantity of nutrients and essential oils given in the recipe, as the cream already contains a proportion of these.

Light Body Lotion with Jasmine and Bergamot

This lotion is ideal to use in the winter months as an all over body lotion. The fragrance is floral and uplifting, and the light lotion is easily and quickly absorbed by the skin. Either use a light lotion base or thin down some Almond Oil and Rosehip Seed Cream (page 48) with orange flower water. Don't forget to halve the quantities in this recipe if you use thinned down face cream. Oat plant milk is a gentle, natural moisturizer that is easily absorbed by the skin.

what's in it?
6½ tbsp (100 ml) light lotion base

1 tsp (5 ml) cornflower water

4 tbsp (50 ml) oat plant milk

15 drops jasmine

5 drops petitgrain

10 drops bergamot

how's it made?
1 Pour the lotion base into a 8 or 10 oz (200 or 250 ml) glass bottle.

2 Pour the cornflower water into the bottle, put on the cap, and shake vigorously to thoroughly mix the ingredients. Then pour in the oat plant milk and shake well.

3 Carefully add the essential oils into the bottle, one by one, then put on the cap and shake vigorously.

4 Label the bottle and the Light Body Lotion with Jasmine and Bergamot is ready to use.

After Sun Body Lotion

This lotion is also good for dry and sensitive skin in addition to use after sunbathing. After the skin has been exposed to the sun, it tends to soak up lotions very quickly. It's important to use this lotion sparingly to prevent overloading your body with too much essential oil. If your skin needs more lotion after one application, use plain body lotion base, and return to using the After Sun lotion the following day.

what's in it?

¾ cup (150 ml) rich lotion base	5 drops neroli
1 tsp (5 ml) rose water	5 drops lavender
1 tsp (5 ml) infused carrot seed oil	5 drops sandalwood
10 drops chamomile	5 drops frankincense

how's it made?

1 Pour the lotion base into a 8 or 10 oz (200 or 250 ml) glass bottle.

2 Pour the rose water into the bottle, put on the cap, and shake vigorously to thoroughly mix the ingredients. Then add the carrot oil and shake well.

3 Carefully add the essential oils into the bottle, one by one, then put on the cap and shake vigorously.

4 Label the bottle and the After Sun Body Lotion is now ready to use.

Rich Body Lotion with Avocado Oil

Powerful and revitalizing essential oils combine with a rich lotion base and avocado oil to make an effective and luxurious body lotion. The fragrance is sumptuous and exotic, and this is a wonderful lotion to use after an evening bath for a romantic evening. This lotion is suitable for all skin types and works especially well on mature and dry skin.

what's in it?

¾ cup (150 ml) rich lotion base	10 drops patchouli
1 teaspoon Monoi de Tahiti	5 drops neroli
1 tsp (5 ml) rose water	5 drops rose
1 tsp (5 ml) avocado oil	5 drops vanilla
	5 drops orange

how's it made?

1 Pour the lotion base into a 8 or 10 oz (200 or 250 ml) glass bottle. Warm the bottle in a mug of hot water. Melt the Monoi de Tahiti in a small dish in the microwave and add to the bottle. Shake well.

2 Pour the rose water into the bottle, put on the cap, and shake vigorously to thoroughly mix the ingredients. Then add the avocado oil and shake well.

3 Carefully add the essential oils into the bottle, one by one, then put on the cap and shake vigorously.

4 Label the bottle and the Rich Body Lotion with Avocado Oil is now ready to use.

Did You Know? *Avocado oil is rich and nourishing and works especially well on mature and dry skin, helping to prevent wrinkles.*

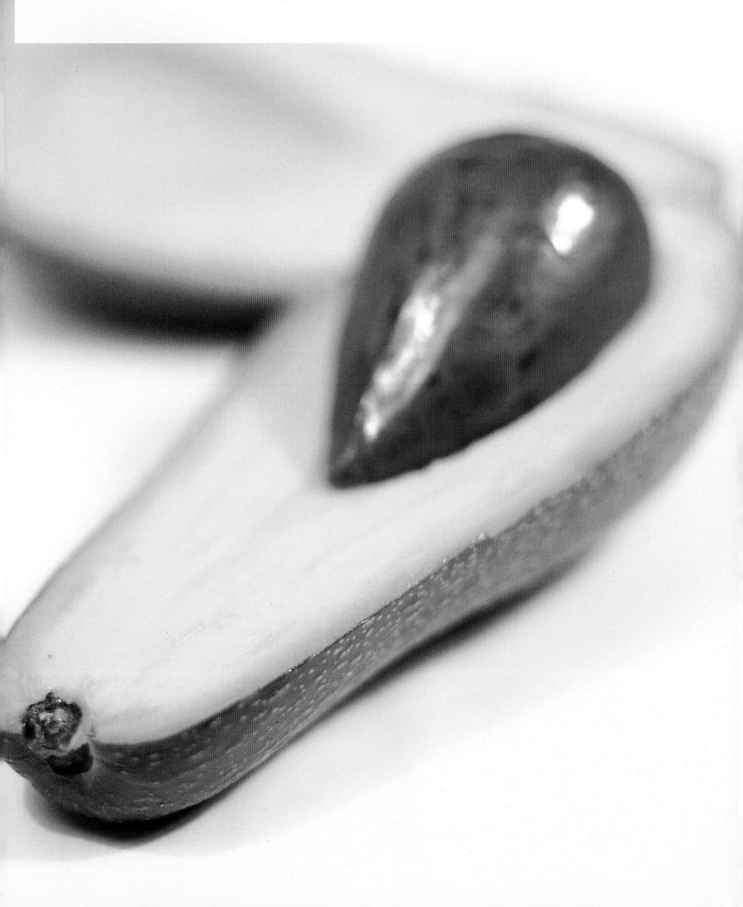

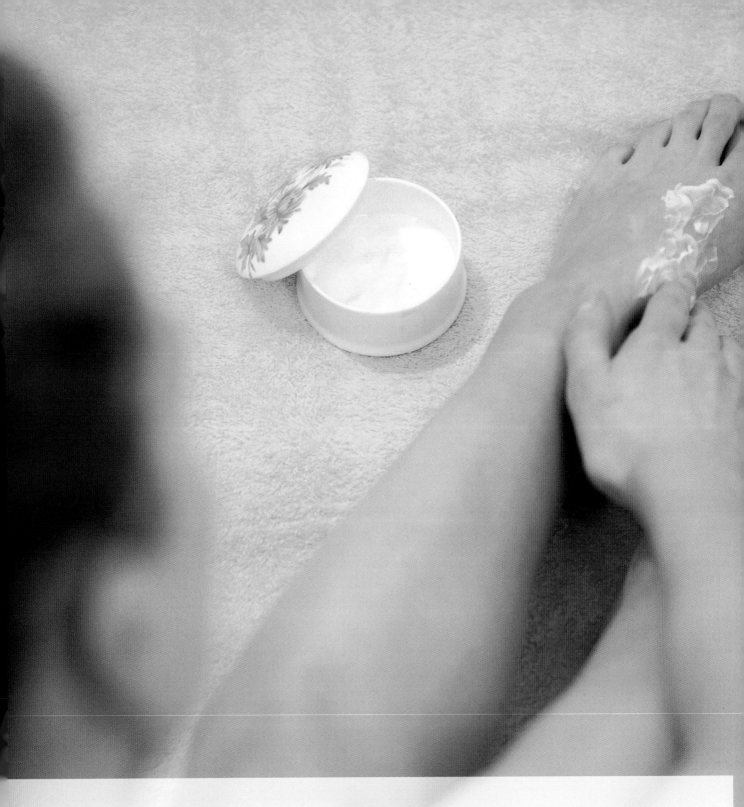

Tip: *This home pedicure keeps your feet looking good as well as feeling good. Do it once a week for a month before going on your summer vacation and your feet will look great.*

Peppermint Foot Lotion

Our feet do a hard job for us every day, carrying our body weight and frequently walking long distances. This stimulating and refreshing foot lotion is a great way to revive and rejuvenate tired feet. Soak your feet in a bowl of hot water for ten minutes, then scrub off any dead skin. Gently rub your feet with this lotion and they will feel wonderful afterwards!

what's in it?

¾ cup (150 ml) light lotion base

1 tsp (5 ml) orange flower water

15 drops peppermint

5 drops lemon

5 drops cypress

5 drops juniper

how's it made?

1 Pour the lotion base into a 8 or 10 oz (200 or 250 ml) glass bottle.

2 Pour the orange flower water into the bottle, put on the cap, and shake vigorously to thoroughly mix the ingredients.

3 Carefully add the essential oils into the bottle, one by one, then put on the cap and shake vigorously.

4 Label the bottle and the Peppermint Foot Lotion is now ready to use.

Lip Balms

Lip balms are indispensable in the winter to avoid sore, chapped lips. Although lipsticks can protect your lips to some extent, many people prefer lip balms, as they are usually made without the use of animal fats. It also means you can protect your lips without coloring them as well.

Homemade lip balms are really effective. Using a natural, organic base and infused oils, essential oils, and beeswax, you can create nourishing lip balms that will protect your lips against the drying effects of cold, wind, and central heating.

The following recipes make enough to fill five small, ½ oz (15 gm) glass jars. You could also use ornamental ceramic pots, if you prefer. Avoid using one large jar as the lip balm will keep better in smaller containers.

Aniseed and Lemon Lip Balm

This is a tangy, refreshing lip balm that leaves a fresh, clean taste on your lips. The base of almond and apricot oils gently lubricates and moisturizes the lips, while the vitamin E is good for regenerating the lips' delicate skin.

what's in it?

- 5 drops yellow color base (see step 1)
- 2 tbsp (30 ml) calendula oil
- 4 tbsp (50 ml) sweet almond oil
- 2 tbsp (25 ml) apricot kernel oil
- 1 drop liquid honey
- 1 tbsp (12 gm) beeswax pellets
- 2 vitamin E capsules
- 2 drops aniseed
- 3 drops lemon

how's it made?

1 Make the yellow color base by adding one teaspoon of ground turmeric to one tablespoon of sunflower oil in a small cup. Heat over boiling water or in a microwave until it bubbles, then remove from heat and pour into a dropper bottle.

2 Prepare a double boiler (one saucepan that fits inside another) by filling the bottom half with hot water and heating to a gentle simmer.

3 Measure out the base oils, one by one, and pour into the top half of the boiler.

4 Add the honey, beeswax pellets, and yellow color base. Stir gently to mix the ingredients.

5 As the beeswax is melting, prick open the vitamin E capsules and squeeze the contents into the oils.

6 Once the beeswax has fully melted remove from the heat. Drop in the aniseed and lemon and stir to mix them in thoroughly.

7 Pour into small glass jars or ceramic pots, and let cool for half an hour or until set. The lip balm is ready to use.

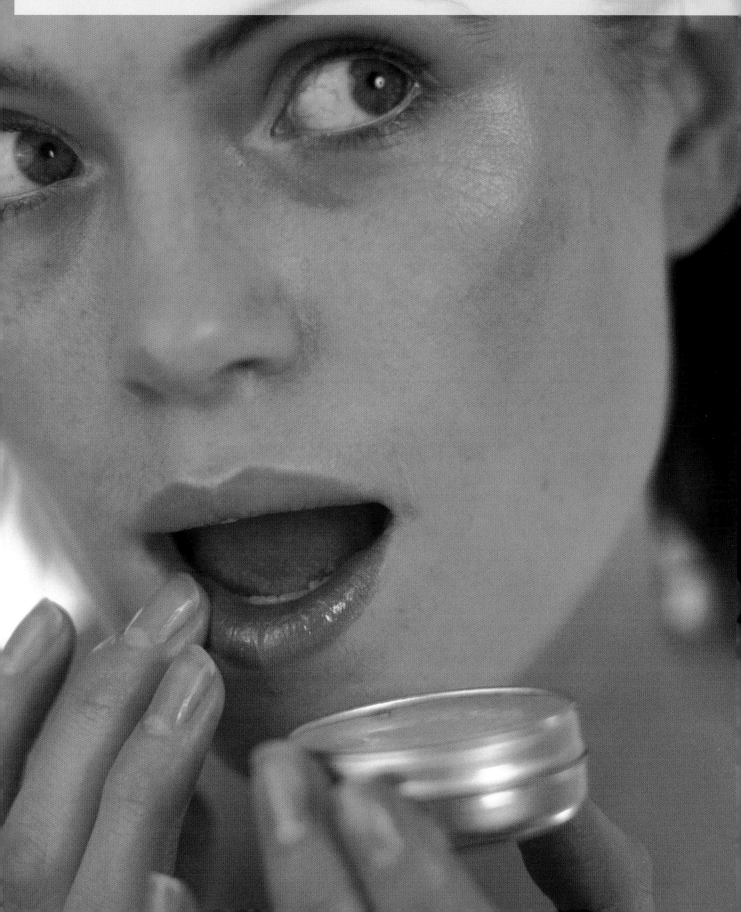

Tip: *The yellow color base gives the impression of lemon, but you could use a brown color base if you prefer, as this gives the impression of aniseed. Alternatively, you can omit the color altogether.*

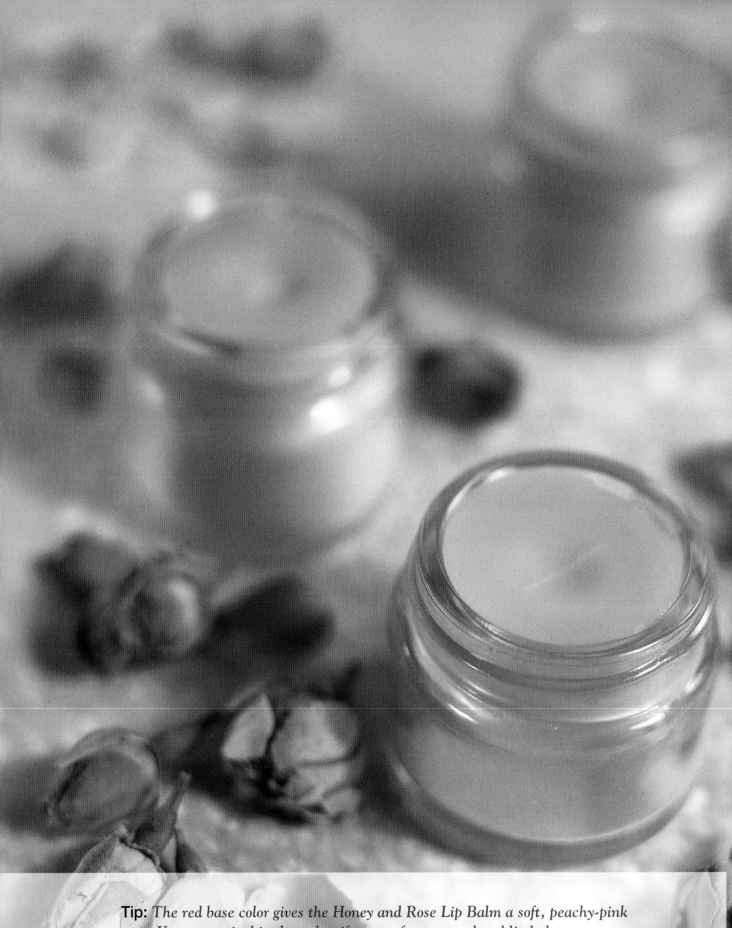

Tip: *The red base color gives the Honey and Rose Lip Balm a soft, peachy-pink tone. You can omit this altogether if you prefer an uncolored lip balm, or increase the number of drops to achieve a deeper shade of color.*

Honey and Rose Lip Balm

The delicate smell of roses combines with the sweetness of honey to make a truly scrumptious and luxurious lip balm. The use of healing calendula oil soothes and heals chapped lips, while the rosehip oil keeps the lips smooth and moisturized.

what's in it?

5 drops red color base (see step 1)	1 drop liquid honey
1 tbsp (15 ml) rosehip seed oil	1 tbsp (12 gm) beeswax pellets
1 tbsp (15 ml) calendula oil	2 vitamin E capsules
5 tbsp (75 ml) sweet almond oil	5 drops rose

how's it made?

1 Make the red color base by adding one teaspoon of ground alkanet root to one tablespoon of sunflower oil in a small cup. Heat over boiling water or in a microwave until it bubbles, then remove from heat and pour into a dropper bottle.

2 Prepare the double boiler (one saucepan that fits inside another) by filling the bottom half with hot water and heating to a gentle simmer.

3 Measure out the base oils, one by one, and pour into the top half of the boiler.

4 Add the honey, beeswax pellets, and red color base. Stir gently to mix the ingredients.

5 As the beeswax is melting, prick open the vitamin E capsules and squeeze the contents into the oils.

6 Once the beeswax has fully melted, remove from the heat. Drop in the rose and stir to mix it in thoroughly.

7 Pour into small glass jars or ceramic pots, and let cool for half an hour or until set. The lip balm is ready to use.

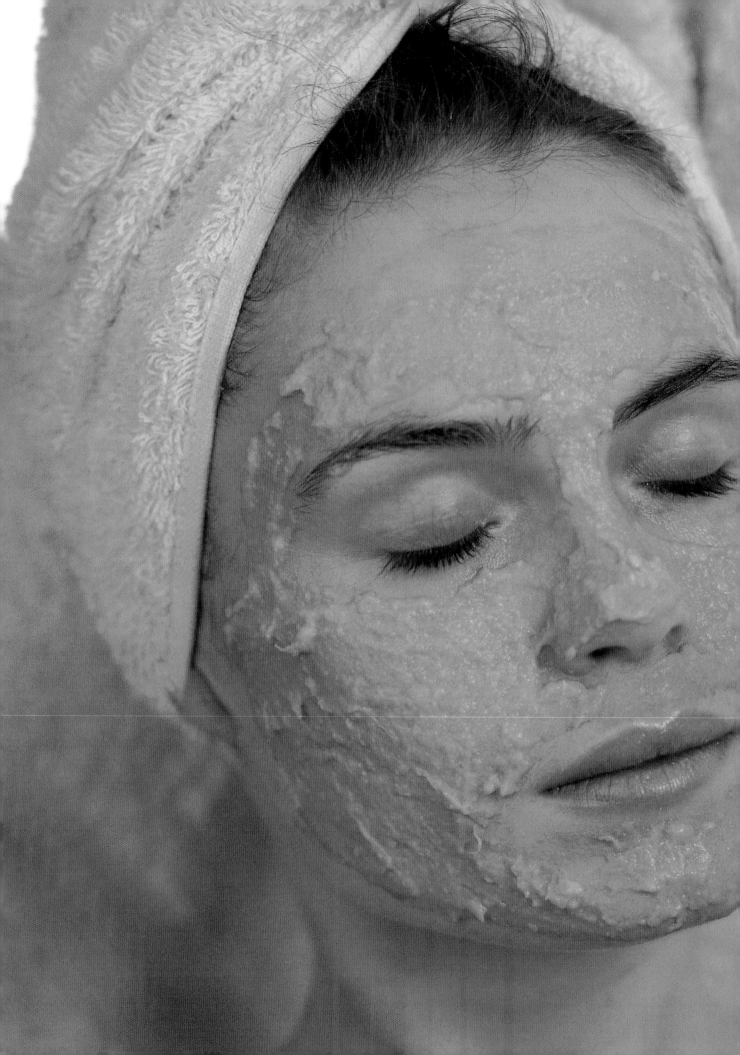

Chapter Four

Face Masks and Rejuvenating Treatments

"Dull skin, rough hands, and so forth will not inspire confidence."
–Patricia Davis, *author and aromatherapist*

Organic Beauty Treatments

Skin creams and lotions moisturize the skin and can be used daily as part of a skin-care regime alongside cleansers and toners. However, we need specialized rejuvenating treatments once a week or month to keep our face and body looking and feeling in tip-top condition. In this chapter, you will find recipes for face masks, exfoliating scrubs, and a luxurious and rejuvenating bath milk.

Face masks are a major rejuvenating treatment. They are applied to the face and the neck—take care to avoid the eyes, the surrounding delicate skin, and the mouth—and left for ten or fifteen minutes to do their work. Masks serve one of several purposes, depending on the ingredients used. Some masks are enriching and nourishing, feeding and hydrating the skin. Ingredients for these masks include honey, almond, and avocado.

Sadly, face masks alone won't transform your skin into the dewy complexion of a model! So, it is a good idea to spend a day detoxifying from the inside as well as from the outside. If you choose a day when you don't have to work, you can really rest and revitalize your whole system. During the day, avoid all caffeine, salt, chemical additives, and alcohol. Drink herb teas and a lot of spring water. Eat a lot of fruit—melons and grapes are especially good for detoxifying your system. Make a simple vegetable soup for lunch and in the evening steam some organic vegetables and serve them with organic brown rice.

As well as applying one of the face masks that follow, you can thoroughly cleanse and tone your face beforehand and give yourself a face massage. In one teaspoon of almond oil put a single drop of rose, jasmine, or neroli. Massage this gently into your face and neck, avoiding the eyes and mouth. After the massage, rest for five minutes with a warm, damp cloth over your face. Then, apply your chosen face mask and rest for ten or fifteen minutes before washing it off with warm water.

Skin benefits from regular exfoliation, and a recipe for a body scrub is also provided. This is important in the spring, as your body has been swathed in thick clothes and subject to the drying effects of wind and central heating. However, regular exfoliation year round keeps the skin in good condition, vibrantly glowing, and healthy.

The feet benefit from a coarser scrub than the rest of the body as the skin is thicker. Use a handful of sea salt, and rub firmly in circular movements, targeting the areas of hard skin. Wash off the salt with warm water and then apply the Peppermint Foot Lotion or Coconut Oil Hand Cream (see pages 59 and 52, respectively), or give yourself a foot massage with a few drops of an essential oil of your choice mixed into a teaspoon of almond oil.

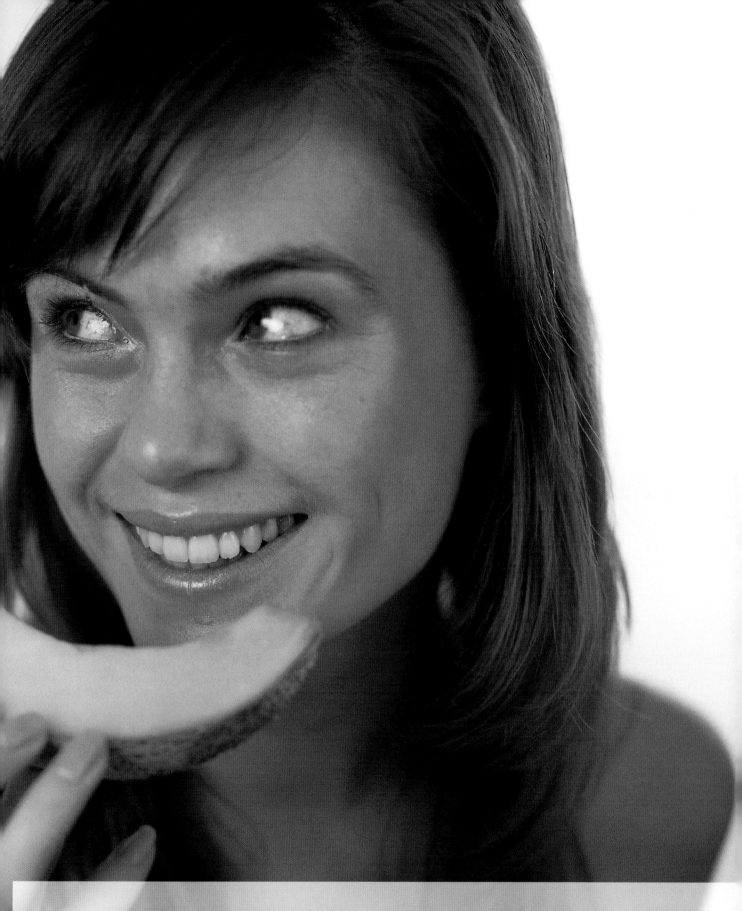

Tip: *While face masks will help nourish your skin, you should also take time to detoxify from the inside as well. To this end, make sure you eat lots of organic fresh fruit, especially melons.*

Face Masks

Following are recipes for face masks, including a deep cleansing mask with green clay and a skin nourishing mask with almonds and honey. Check the condition of your skin, as well as your skin type, before choosing which face mask to use. Does your skin look dull and need a deep cleanse? Or perhaps your skin feels tired and dry and needs a nourishing mask?

Homemade face masks are fun but messy, so make sure you have plenty of old towels around. Also, before you start, decide where you will rest once the mask is applied. Lying down is best, as it stops the mask from slipping off your face. You can make eye pads to cover your eyes. Either soak cotton pads in rose water or keep a couple of cooled, used chamomile tea bags and use these instead.

Avocado Enriching Face Mask

This is one of the simplest face masks to make as it only has one ingredient! Avocado is very nourishing for the skin, and this mask is especially good for mature, wrinkled, and dry skin, although it is suitable for all skin types. Make sure you use a ripe, fresh, organic avocado for the best effect.

what's in it?
1 very ripe, organic avocado

how's it made?

1 Peel the avocado and remove the stone. Chop up the avocado and put it in a small glass bowl.

2 Using a fork, mash the avocado to a creamy pulp, making sure you break down any lumps.

3 Apply the avocado mask immediately to a cleansed face, and rest for ten minutes.

4 Finally, wash off the mask with warm water and apply a toner and moisturizer.

Honey and Almond Moisturizing Face Mask

The combination of honey and ground almonds makes this mask smell good enough to eat! Although it feels very sticky, and takes a lot of washing off, this is nonetheless a wonderful face mask, and worth the effort. The honey and almond moisturizing face mask is particularly good for mature, sensitive, or dry skin, but is suitable for all skin types.

what's in it?

1 large tsp honey

1 tbsp ground almonds

Enough warm water to mix to a spreadable paste

how's it made?

1 Warm the honey in a small bowl immersed in hot water until it becomes liquid.

2 Put the ground almonds into another small bowl. Add the melted honey and mix well, adding a little warm water to obtain a spreadable consistency.

3 Immediately apply the mask to a cleansed face and rest for ten to fifteen minutes.

4 Finally, wash off the mask with warm water and apply a toner and moisturizer.

Yogurt and Oatmeal Deep Cleansing Face Mask

Yogurt has been used for centuries for its health giving properties. Here, live, organic yogurt is mixed with finely ground oatmeal and a little honey for an all purpose face mask. This face mask is suited to all skin types, and is both cleansing and rejuvenating. If you have any doubt about which face mask to use, this is the one to go for.

what's in it?

1 tbsp finely ground oatmeal

1 tbsp live, organic yogurt

1 small tsp honey

how's it made?

1 Place the oatmeal in a bowl. Add the yogurt and mix to a spreadable consistency.

2 Warm the honey in a small glass bowl. Pour into the yogurt and oatmeal mixture and blend the ingredients thoroughly.

3 Immediately apply the yogurt and oatmeal mask to a cleansed face and rest for ten to fifteen minutes.

4 Finally, wash off the mask with warm water and apply a toner and moisturizer.

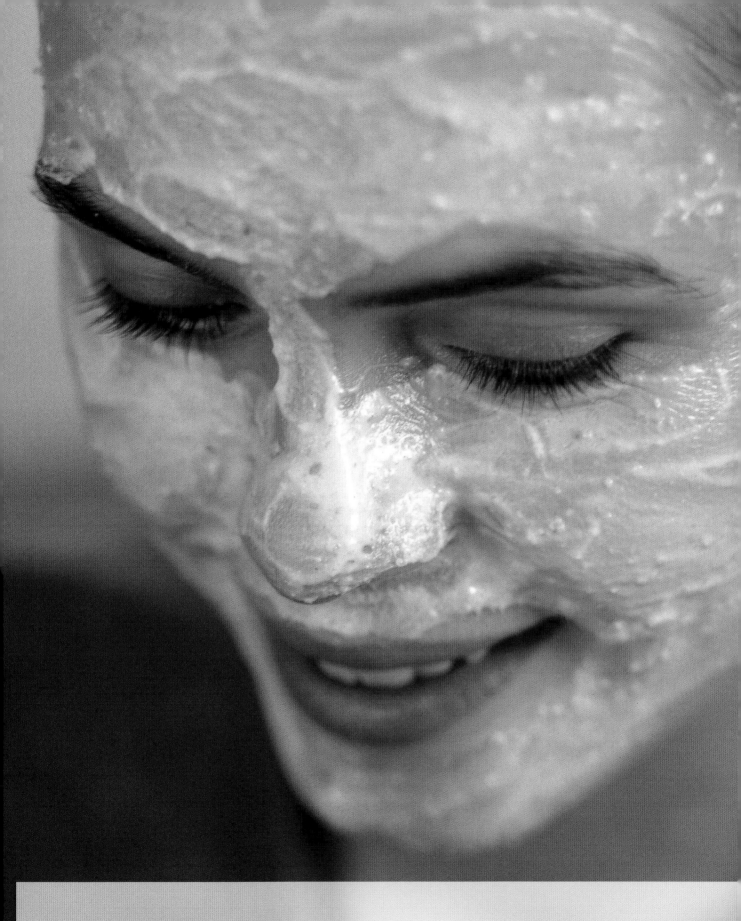

Did You Know? *Yogurt has a softening effect on the skin and a very mild bleaching action, helping to dispel skin blemishes.*

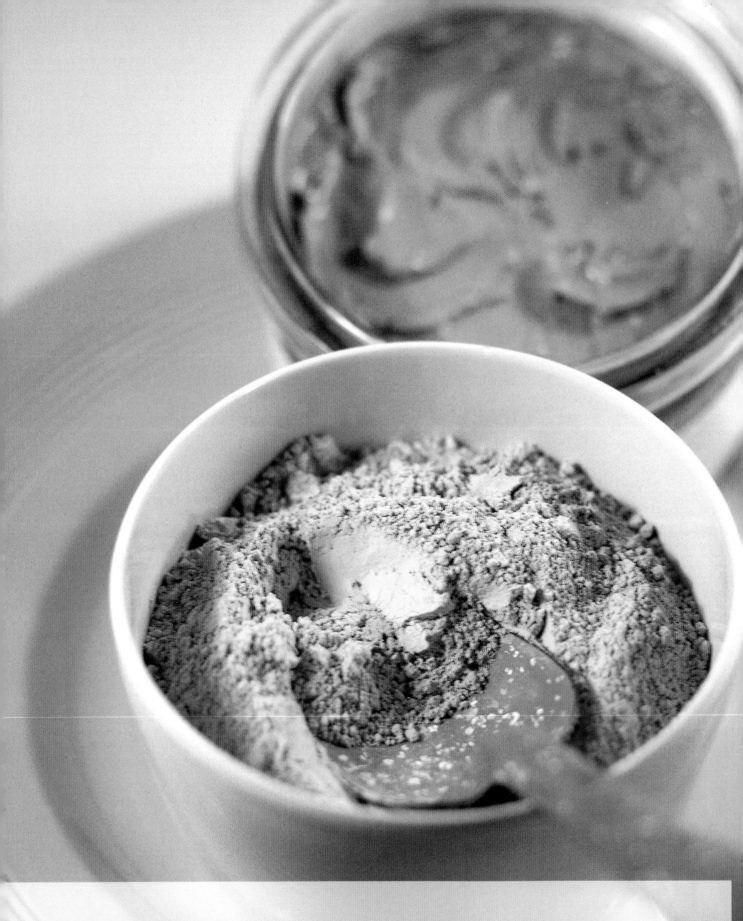

Tip: *If you have dry skin but would like to use the green clay mask, double the quantity of the apricot oil.*

Green Clay Purifying Mask

Green clay is also known as bentonite, and is the most commonly used clay in face masks. It has a slippery feel and can absorb large quantities of water. This mask is used to draw out excess sebum, toxins, and dirt from deep down in the skin and is best suited to oily skin. Green clay stabilizes the production of sebum and deeply cleanses the skin.

what's in it?

1 tsp apricot kernel oil
2 drops palmarosa
1 tbsp green clay
Enough warm water to mix to a spreadable paste

how's it made?

1 Mix the apricot oil and the palmarosa together in small dish.

2 Put the green clay in a small bowl. Add the apricot oil mixture and stir. Add just enough warm water to make a spreadable paste, and work the mixture thoroughly to incorporate all the ingredients.

3 Immediately apply the mask to a cleansed face and rest for ten to fifteen minutes. The mask will tighten slightly as the water evaporates and may feel a little strange. Don't worry; it's just the mask doing its work.

4 Finally, wash off the mask with warm water and apply a toner and moisturizer.

Rejuvenating Treatments

These rejuvenating treatments are designed to restore the skin's natural bloom. The body scrub achieves this effect by exfoliation, the removal of the skin's surface of dead skin cells, revealing the fresh new skin underneath. Exfoliation also stimulates the circulation, bringing more blood and nutrients to the skin and carrying away the toxins. Ideally, you should have a body scrub once a month, but even an occasional scrub will leave you with lovely skin for a while.

The bath milk and face oil are luxurious moisturizing treatments that deeply penetrate the skin with enriching, nourishing oils that help the skin retain its natural elasticity and restore its smooth, glowing appearance. The nutrients and oils combine to create rejuvenating treatments that leave you feeling invigorated and give you silky smooth skin that also smells divine. These two treatments are easier to make up and use than the body scrub, and you could aim to do them once a week.

Rejuvenating Rose Bath Milk

Bathing in milk is an ancient beauty treatment, first popularized by Cleopatra, who took weekly baths of assess' milk. These days, there are available store-bought bath milks already fragranced, and base bath milks that you can customize with essential oils. This recipe also contains the nourishing natural moisturizing properties of almonds and the rejuvenating effect of pure, organic rose oil.

what's in it?
2 tsp (10 gm) ground almonds
6½ tbsp (100 ml) rose water
6½ tbsp (100 ml) bath milk base
50 drops rose

how's it made?

1 Place the ground almonds and rose water in a blender. Blend for a couple of minutes. Let the mixture stand for a few minutes, then blend again for a couple of minutes. Repeat once more.

2 Strain the rose and almond milk through fine muslin into a container, then pour into a 9 oz (250 ml) glass bottle.

3 Add the bath milk base and shake well. Carefully count in the drops of rose, and shake well so all the ingredients are thoroughly blended.

4 Label the bottle and the Rejuvenating Rose Bath Milk is ready to use. For each bath, pour in one or two tablespoons of bath milk.

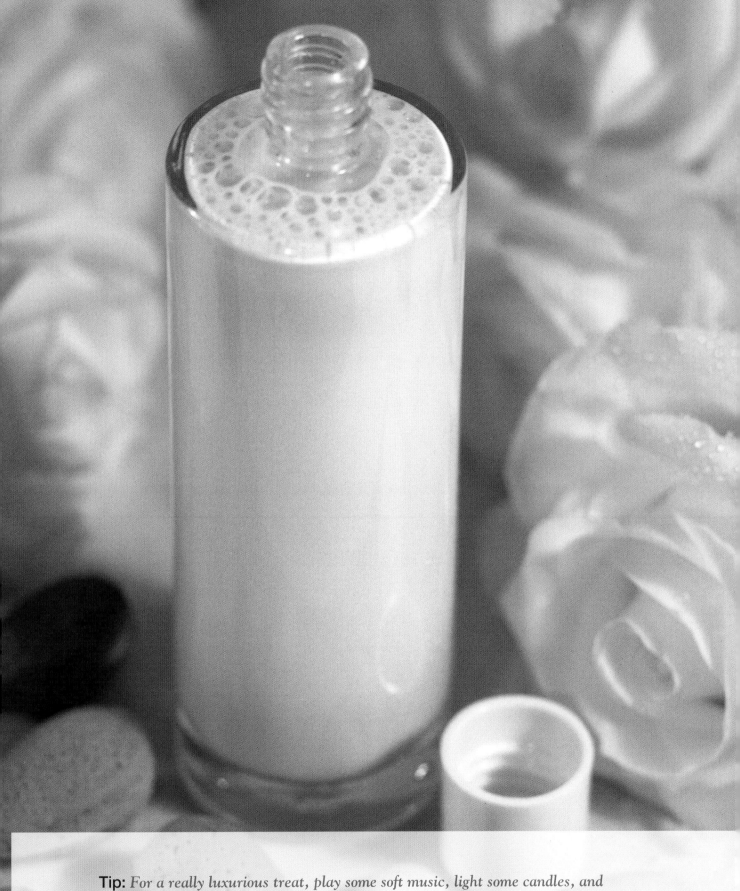

Tip: *For a really luxurious treat, play some soft music, light some candles, and have a glass of something bubbly as you lie back in the fragrant, healing water.*

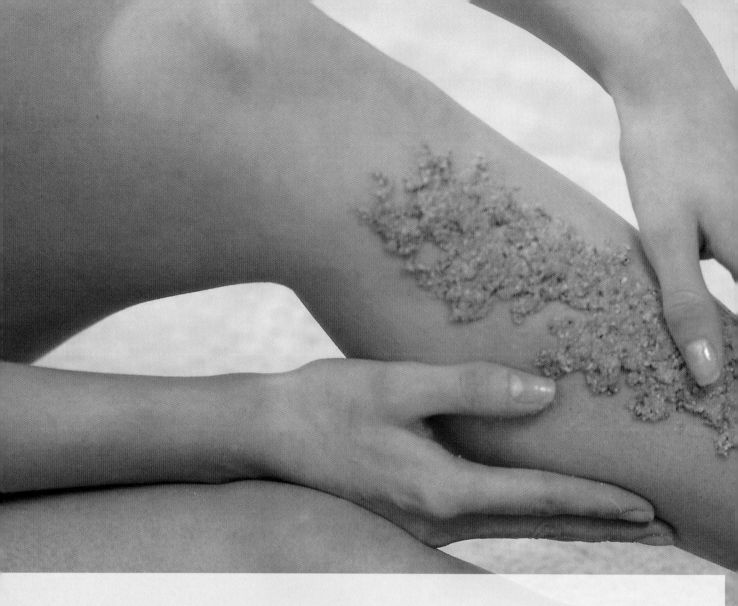

Tip: *You could try doing the Rejuvenating, Exfoliating Body Scrub with your partner or friend, as it is easier to scrub someone else than to scrub yourself, though it is fine to do by yourself too. It's best to do the body scrub standing in the bath, as it's a messy procedure.*

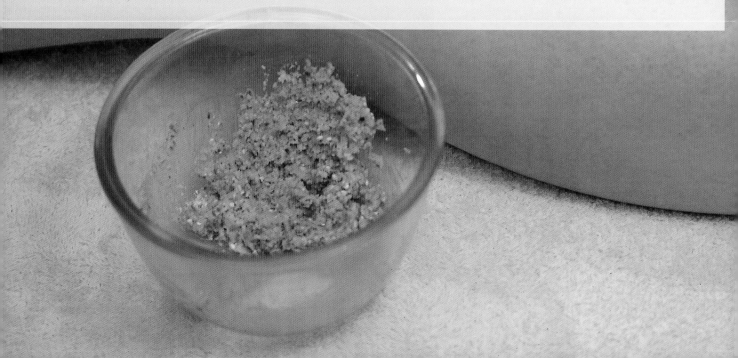

Rejuvenating, Exfoliating Body Scrub

This rejuvenating treatment is based on a traditional Indian body scrub for brides. The bride is scrubbed all over with a traditional mixture of finely ground grains, fruit peels, spices, and oils, and then she is massaged with sweet smelling oils. This is performed daily for ten days, so at the wedding she looks wonderful with smooth, sweet smelling skin. Using this body scrub will leave you with glowing skin.

what's in it?

2 tbsp fine ground oatmeal

2 tbsp ground almonds

1 tsp dried, finely ground orange peel

1 tsp rosehip granules

5 drops jasmine

Enough warm water to moisten the mixture

how's it made?

1 Place all the dried ingredients in a large bowl and mix thoroughly.

2 Add the jasmine and a little warm water to make a fine, crumbly mixture. Don't use too much water or you will end up with a sticky mess.

3 Stand in the bathtub or on a towel spread over the floor. Take a small handful of the body scrub and scrub vigorously with circular movements all over the body. Be systematic; do the legs and arms first as they are easiest, and then do as much of the rest of your body as you can reach.

4 The scrub dries quickly, and most of it will fall off your body. When you have finished, use a soft body brush to brush off any leftover crumbs.

Rejuvenating Face Oil

Although this face oil takes a little longer than a face cream to be absorbed into the skin, using this rejuvenating face oil once a week will literally feed your face with exceptional nutrients. Make sure you have thoroughly cleansed and toned your face before applying the face oil. You don't need a moisturizing face cream, as the face oil itself is deeply moisturizing.

what's in it?

1 tbsp (10 ml) kukui nut oil	3 evening primrose oil
1 tbsp (10 ml) jojoba oil	capsules
1 tbsp (10 ml) apricot	4 drops rose
kernel oil	3 drops neroli
1 tsp (5 ml) almond oil	3 drops jasmine
1 tsp (5 ml) avocado oil	3 drops frankincense
1 tbsp (10 ml) rosehip oil	2 drops sandalwood

how's it made?

1 Carefully measure out and pour all the base oils into a 2 or 3 oz (75 or 100 ml) dark glass bottle. Shake well.

2 With a pin, prick open the capsules of evening primrose oil and squeeze in to the bottle.

3 Carefully add in the essential oils, one by one. Shake the bottle well.

4 Label the bottle. The Rejuvenating Face Oil is ready to use.

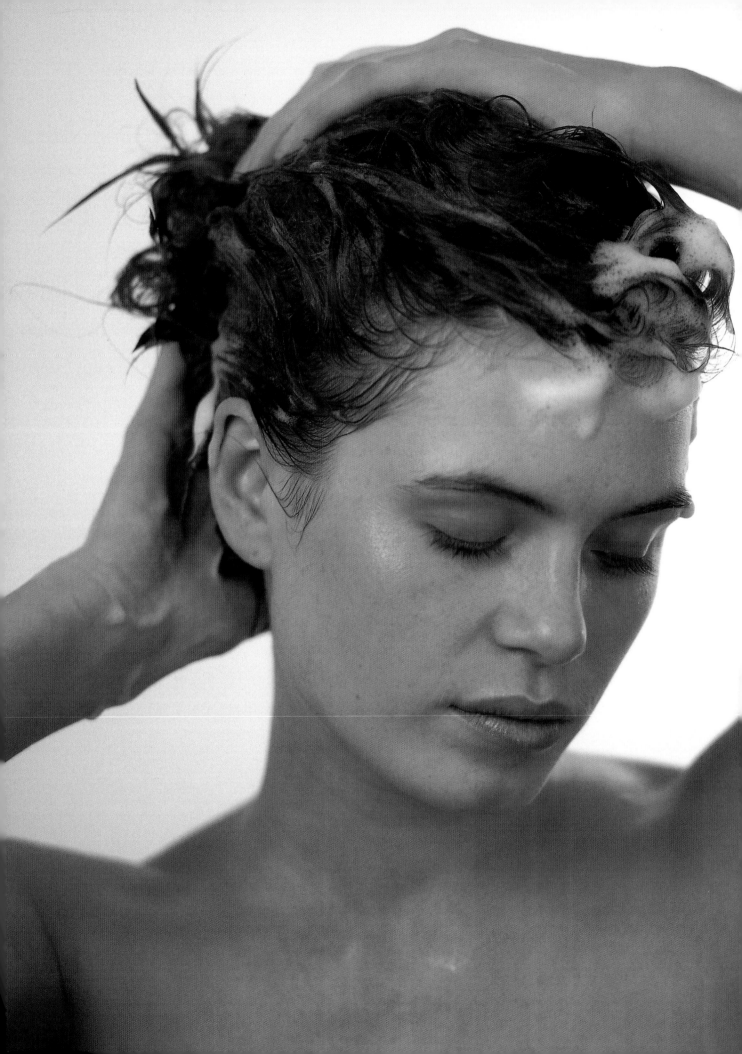

Chapter Five

Hair Shampoos and Conditioners

"Synthetics have intruded upon all areas of our lives—we need only read the back of our shampoo bottle for an example."
—Susan Miller Cavitch, *natural soap maker and author*

Homemade Hair Care

Our hair is mainly composed of a protein called keratin, which also forms our fingernails and the outer layer of our skin. Keratin is actually dead tissue, produced as the living cells—including those in the hair root, or follicle—die and are replaced by new cells. This means the health of your hair depends on the health of the hair follicles, from which the hair grows. The hair follicles depend on a good supply of oxygen from the surrounding blood vessels, so to keep your hair in good condition you need to stimulate circulation in the scalp by regular head massage.

You already do a little massage when you shampoo your hair, and using a hair brush is also stimulating for the scalp. However, if you would like to improve the condition of your hair, try doing a scalp massage daily for five minutes or so. Use small, firm, circular movements with your fingertips, and make sure you move the scalp itself, so you are not just massaging your hair.

No oil is required for this scalp massage, but doing a massage with oil once a week will condition the hair and scalp, although you will have to wash your hair afterward. Take one teaspoon of warmed almond oil and add three drops of essential oil. Dip your fingers frequently into this mixture as you do the scalp massage. If you have dark hair, use rosemary; for fair hair, use chamomile; and if you suffer from dandruff, use sandalwood, lavender, or bergamot.

Our hair benefits from natural, organic, plant-based products as much as our face and body. Many store-bought shampoos are harsh, and although they leave the hair clean, they strip off the natural coating of sebum. Sebum is our own natural moisturizer; an oily wax produced by glands in the body and in the hair follicles.

Shampoo and conditioner bases can be bought from one of the suppliers listed on pages 124–125. These shampoos and conditioners are made from natural plant material—often organic—and contain no chemical additives. This means they are exceptionally mild, and leave the hair clean but not stripped completely of sebum.

The mildness of these plant-based hair-care products also means the scalp is cared for and not aggravated by harsh cleansers or chemicals. If you are prone to an itchy or flakey scalp, switching to your own homemade shampoos and conditioners could well relieve you of these unpleasant symptoms. After a few weeks of using these mild, natural hair treatments you are likely to have a healthy scalp and soft, glossy hair.

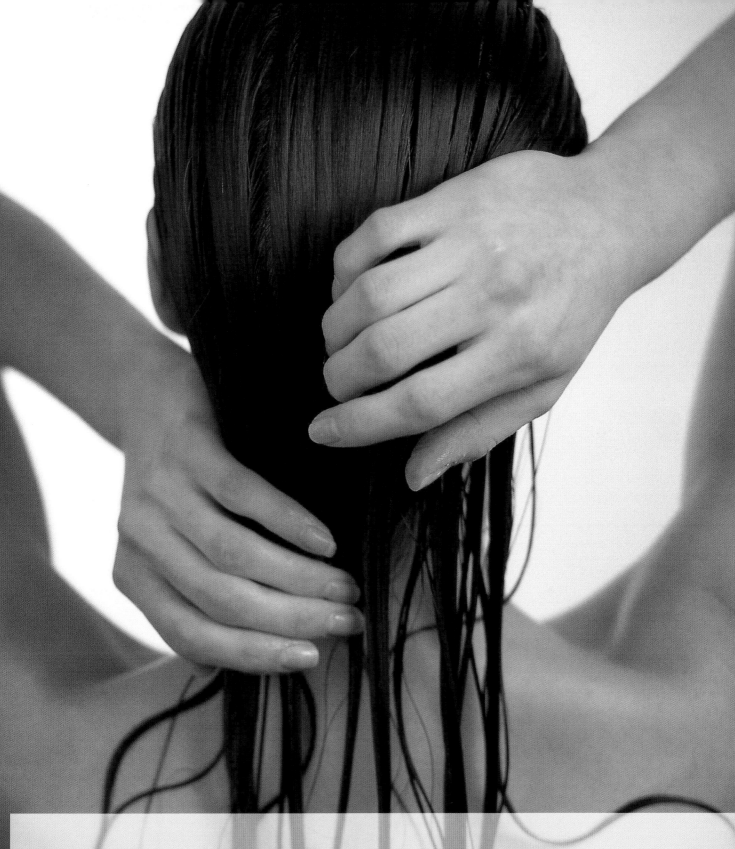

Did You Know? When we brush our hair, we spread the sebum along the individual hair shafts, and it is this that keeps our hair shiny, smooth, and glossy. Without the protective coating of sebum, the hair becomes dull, brittle, and lifeless, and the hair ends are prone to splitting.

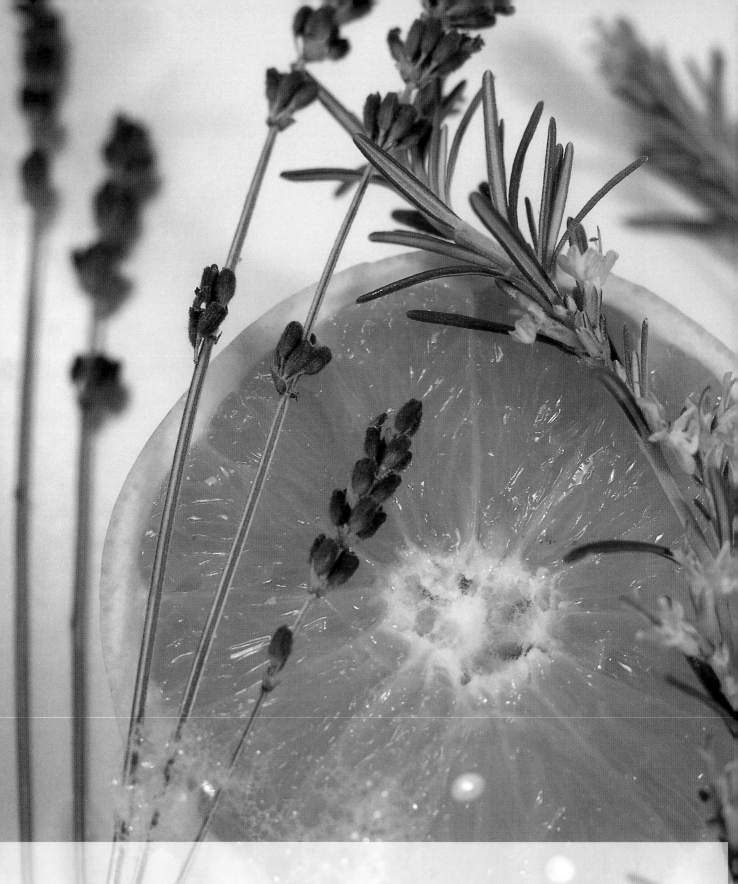

Did You Know? When citrus oils are blended into shampoo, they leave your hair smelling incredibly fresh and clean.

Shampoos

Caring for your hair and scalp is easy when you use mild shampoos enriched and perfumed with essential oils. Buying your shampoo base from a supplier of natural cosmetic products ensures you will get a high-quality, mild, natural, plant-based shampoo. Instead of harsh detergents and chemicals, the shampoo will be made from mild soaps, together with emulsifiers, nutrients, and so forth. These combine to make a shampoo gentle enough for even the most sensitive skin and hair damaged by bleaching or coloring.

Some suppliers offer organic base products, and by adding organic essential oils you will end up with a shampoo that will really care for and protect your hair and scalp in addition to cleaning them thoroughly. Your homemade shampoos are gentle enough to use on a daily basis, if required.

Herbal Shampoo with Pine and Grapefruit

This is a traditional herbal shampoo with the added zing of pine and grapefruit. Lavender and rosemary are often used in shampoos. Lavender calms and soothes the scalp, and rosemary and pine are stimulating, helping bring blood, which is rich in nutrients, to the scalp. Grapefruit has a tonic effect on the skin and scalp and the delightful smell makes a welcome addition to this shampoo. Herbal shampoo is particularly recommended for oily hair but is suitable for all hair types.

what's in it?
6½ tbsp (100 ml) shampoo base
10 drops lavender
10 drops rosemary
5 drops pine
5 drops grapefruit

how's it made?
1 Pour the shampoo base into a glass container with a good pouring spout.

2 Carefully add the essential oils, one by one. Use a glass stirring rod or a chopstick to thoroughly stir the oils.

3 Pour into a glass bottle, plastic squeeze bottle, or pump dispenser using a funnel to avoid spillage.

4 Label the bottle and the herbal shampoo is ready to use.

Chamomile and Geranium Shampoo

This delightful smelling shampoo is a good general shampoo for all hair types but is especially good for dry hair. The combination of chamomile, sandalwood, and geranium provides a restorative effect, helping balance the production of sebum. This shampoo helps restore vitality to dull and lifeless hair, giving a long lasting shine.

what's in it?
6½ tbsp (100 ml) shampoo base
10 drops chamomile
10 drops geranium
5 drops sandalwood
3 drops lemon
2 drops lime

how's it made?
1 Pour the shampoo base into a glass container with a good pouring spout.

2 Carefully add the essential oils, one by one. Use a glass stirring rod or a chopstick to thoroughly stir the oils.

3 Pour into a glass bottle, plastic squeeze bottle, or pump dispenser using a funnel to avoid spillage.

4 Label the bottle and the Chamomile and Geranium Shampoo is ready to use.

Tip: *All essential oils are antiseptic to some extent, but pine is especially effective. Its refreshing and deodorant properties are often used in bathing and cleansing products.*

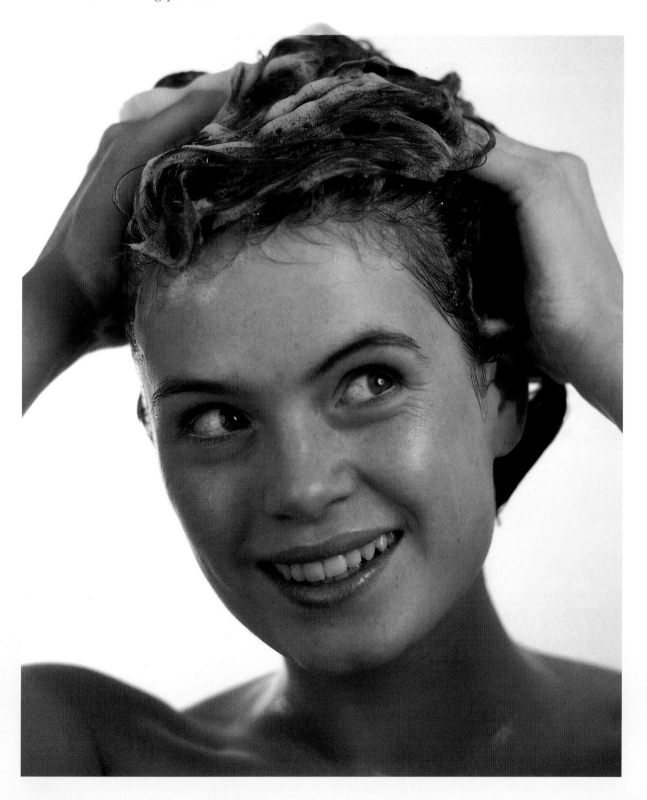

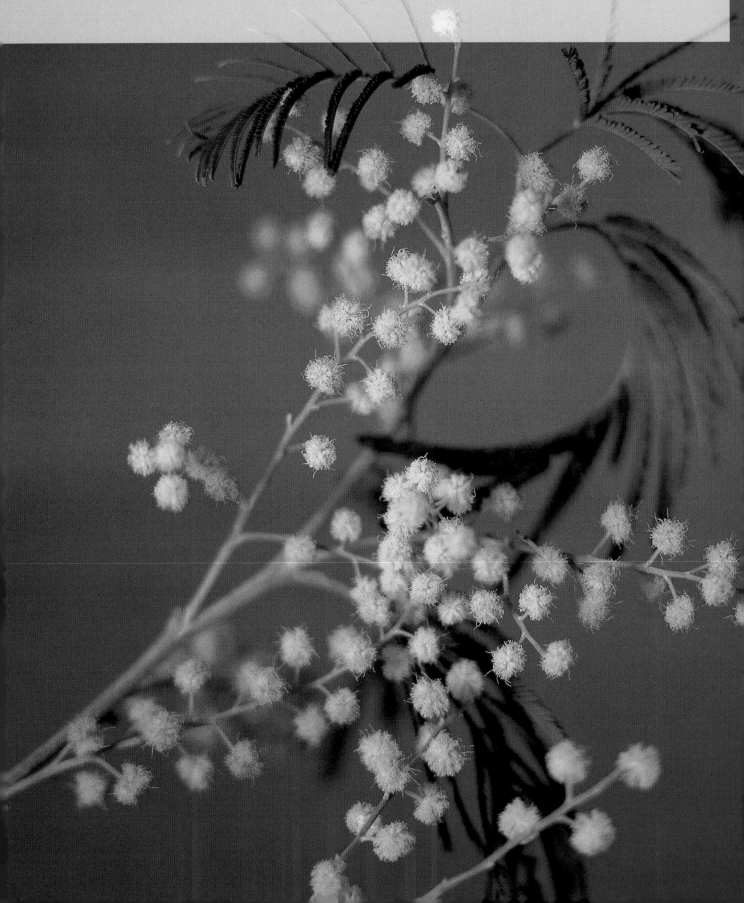

Tip: *The Oat Milk Conditioner with Mimosa and Ylang Ylang is a lovely complement to the Chamomile and Geranium Shampoo on page 84.*

Conditioners and Rinses

After shampooing, it's important to use conditioner to give increased manageability to your hair, leaving it soft and shiny. Conditioners restore vitality and luster and should be used every time you wash your hair. The following conditioners use essential oils to perfume, balance, and nourish your hair. These homemade conditioners make the perfect complement to your homemade shampoos.

Hair rinses are simple and quick to make, and they are effective in restoring the hair's natural pH balance. Hair rinses are also clarifying and remove any last traces of shampoo or conditioner residue that may remain on the hair shaft. This helps make the hair shine. Use a hair rinse once a week after shampooing and using hair conditioner and make sure you rinse it off thoroughly with a lot of cool or tepid water.

Oat Milk Conditioner with Mimosa and Ylang Ylang

This luxuriant conditioner has a sweet, exotic, and floral fragrance and leaves your hair shiny, soft, and manageable. Oat plant milk softens and nourishes the scalp and hair with its mild, gentle moisturizing properties. Oat milk conditioner is especially good for dry, damaged, and colored hair but is suitable for all hair types.

what's in it?
5 tbsp (75 ml) conditioner base

2 tbsp (25 ml) oat plant milk

10 drops ylang ylang

10 drops lavender

5 drops petitgrain

5 drops mimosa

how's it made?

1 Pour the conditioner base into a glass container with a good pouring spout. Add the oat plant milk and stir thoroughly to combine the all the ingredients.

2 Carefully add the essential oils, one by one. Use a glass stirring rod or a chopstick to thoroughly stir in the oils.

3 Pour into a glass bottle, plastic squeeze bottle, or pump dispenser using a funnel to avoid spillage.

4 Label the bottle and the Oat Milk Conditioner is ready to use.

Herbal Conditioner with Clary Sage and Rosewood

Herbs and rosewood combine to make a conditioner that restores a healthy shine and a fresh, clean smell to your hair. Clary sage helps to reduce excessive production of sebum, especially on the scalp. This conditioner is therefore especially suitable for those who have greasy, lank hair. However, unlike commercial conditioners made for greasy hair, this conditioner actively reduces excessive sebum production, which means your hair stays clean longer.

what's in it?

6½ tbsp (100 ml) conditioner base

10 drops clary sage

10 drops rosewood

5 drops rosemary

3 drops lavender

2 drops tea-tree

how's it made?

1 Pour the conditioner base into a glass container with a good pouring spout.

2 Carefully add the essential oils, one by one. Use a glass stirring rod or a chopstick to thoroughly stir in the oils.

3 Pour into a glass bottle, plastic squeeze bottle, or pump dispenser using a funnel to avoid spillage.

4 Label the bottle and the herbal conditioner is ready to use.

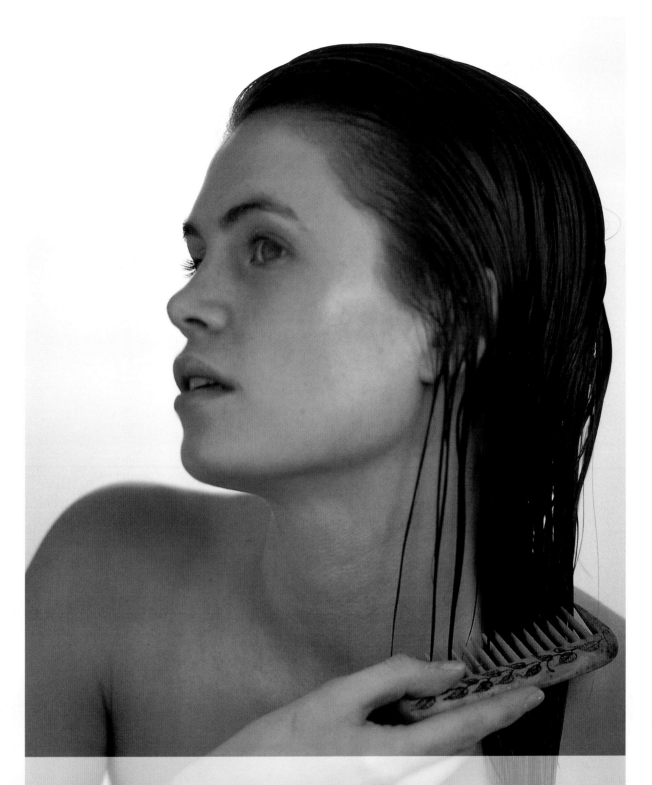

Tip: Herbal Conditioner with Clary Sage and Rosewood helps reduce excessive sebum production. Massage your scalp vigorously with the conditioner before rinsing it off.

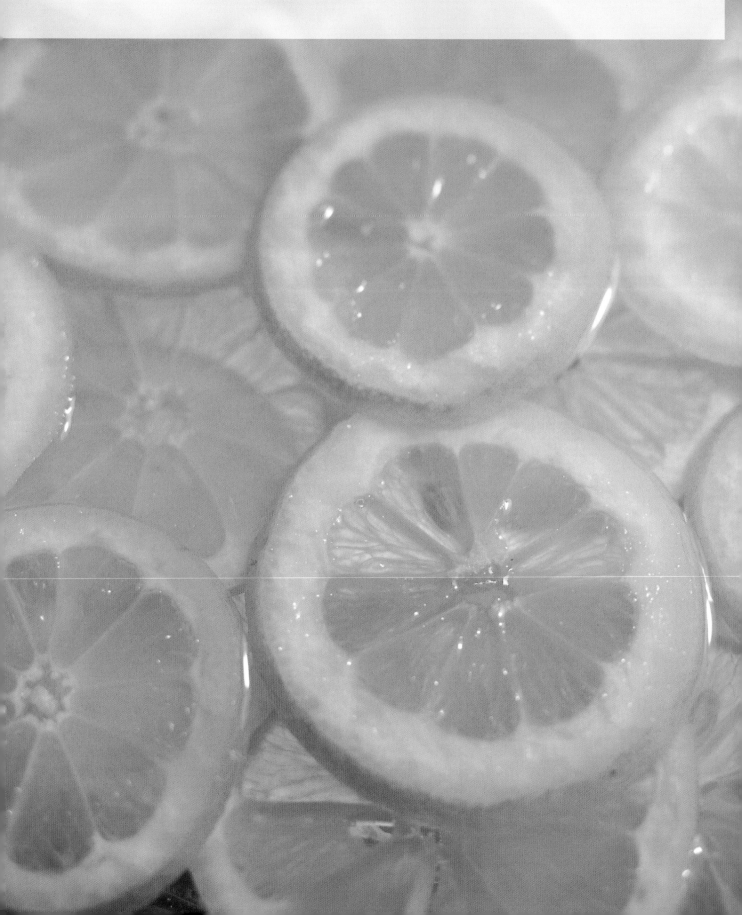

Did You Know? *Lemon has traditionally been used as a hair rinse to brighten dull hair. It's astringent properties also help tone the scalp.*

Apple Cider Vinegar Hair Rinse

Cider vinegar has been used as a hair rinse since the time of our grandmothers, and here apple cider vinegar is used as the base ingredient. Combined with the fresh aroma of orange flower water and petitgrain, this makes a stimulating, clarifying hair rinse. Apple cider vinegar hair rinse is suitable for all hair types, though it works especially well on greasy hair.

what's in it?

1 tsp (5 ml) apple cider vinegar

1 tbsp (10 ml) orange flower water

1 tbsp (10 ml) spring water

3 drops petitgrain

1 drop bergamot

how's it made?

1 Measure the apple cider vinegar into a glass bottle. Add the orange flower water and the spring water. Shake well to combine.

2 Carefully add the essential oils, one by one, and shake well to disperse them.

3 The rinse is ready to use. Slowly pour through your freshly shampooed and conditioned hair. Leave on hair for a couple of minutes.

4 Rinse your hair thoroughly with cool or tepid water.

Lemon and Rosemary Hair Rinse

This recipe uses fresh herbs and lemons—you can easily find fresh organic herbs and citrus fruits. The recipe suggests using rosemary, which is best for dark hair. If you have light hair, substitute chamomile for the rosemary. Parsley is another alternative, and gives your hair a really clean shine.

what's in it?

The juice of one freshly squeezed lemon

1 tsp (5 gm) fresh, finely chopped rosemary, chamomile, or parsley

Enough water to cover the herbs in a small saucepan

how's it made?

1 Squeeze the lemon juice into a glass jug. Put the finely chopped herbs into a saucepan and pour in enough water to cover. Bring to the boil and simmer for five minutes.

2 Strain the mixture through muslin and let the herb infusion cool. Mix 2 tbsp (20 ml) of the herbal infusion into the lemon juice.

3 The rinse is now ready to use. Slowly pour through your freshly shampooed and conditioned hair. Leave on hair for a couple of minutes.

4 Rinse your hair thoroughly with cool or tepid water.

Hot Oil Nourishing Hair Wrap

This treatment is a real treat for your hair. Try to do the hot oil hair wrap once a month. You do need to put aside an evening, but you could combine doing the hair wrap with a body scrub, pedicure, or other beauty treatment. The recipe suggests using almond oil and chamomile, but you can vary the base oil and essential oil according to your hair color and type. Rosemary is good for dark hair. Jojoba oil is good for very dry hair. Sandalwood imparts a lovely, long lasting fragrance, which might be nice for a special occasion.

what's in it?

1 tsp to 1 tbsp (5 to 10 ml) almond oil, depending on
   your hair's length and thickness

3 drops chamomile

how's it made?

1 Warm the almond oil in a small cup or bowl sitting in a larger bowl of hot water. Mix the chamomile in thoroughly.

2 Apply the oil to your hair, making sure you cover every strand. Use the opportunity to give yourself a scalp massage.

3 Wrap your hair in plastic wrap and then cover your head with a hot towel. Replace with another hot towel once the first one has cooled. Leave the oil in for at least two hours.

4 Shampoo your hair at least twice to wash off the oil, then condition your hair as usual. Your hair will feel soft and glossy with a lovely shine.

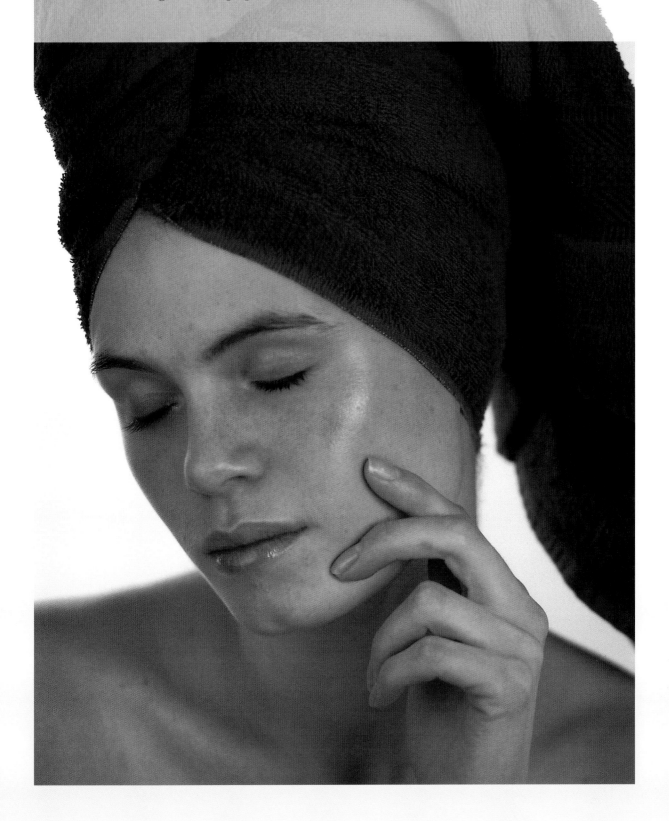

Did You Know? *In India, both men and women routinely use coconut oil as a hair dressing, as it helps protect the hair from the hot sun.*

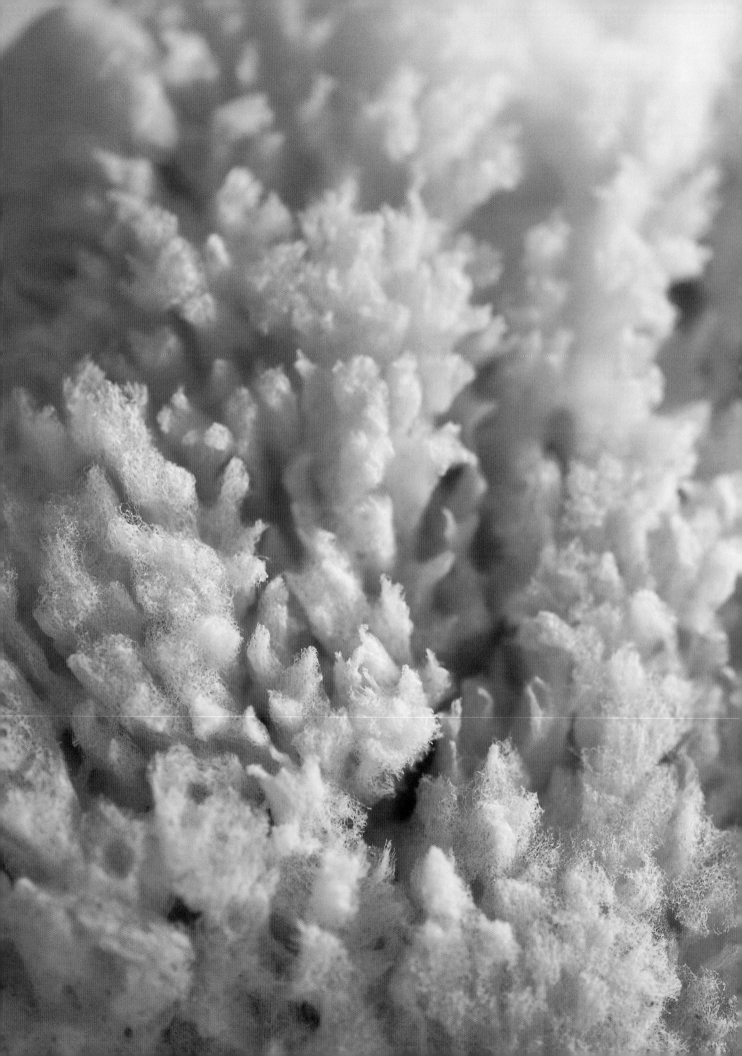

Chapter Six

Naturally Fresh and Clean

"Several essential oils are effective deodorizing agents."
–Patricia Davis, *author and aromatherapist*

Deodorants, Mouthwashes, and Aftershaves

This chapter includes recipes for homemade deodorants, mouthwashes, aftershaves, eye washes, and eye compresses. The recipes are quick and simple to make and lovely to use. All the recipes use only plant-based, natural, and organic ingredients. Essential oils and herbs impart their healing qualities to these cosmetics, and you can rest assured that you are using pure ingredients to keep yourself naturally fresh and clean.

The homemade deodorants have a lovely, clean, fresh aroma. Because they are so gentle on your skin, you can spray them on liberally with no adverse side effects. They will not stain your clothes unlike some commercial deodorants, which can leave white patches on dark clothes or discolor pale-colored ones. The refreshing, uplifting scent will leave you feeling sparkling clean.

However, these homemade deodorants are not as effective or long lasting as many store-bought deodorants. This is because they do not contain any antiperspirant, a substance that actively prevents you from sweating. Our bodies need to sweat, as this is one of the body's ways of cooling down. Sweating also eliminates toxins from the body, so it is a necessary function and should not be discouraged.

The mouthwashes use natural ingredients and essential oils to leave your mouth and gums feeling really fresh and clean. The essential oils also help prevent bacterial growth and discourage and heal mouth ulcers, gum infections, and inflammations such as gingivitis. Using these natural mouthwashes also helps prevent these conditions from arising in the first place and keeps the mouth and gums clean and healthy.

Homemade aftershaves not only are lovely to use but make great gifts for the men in your life. Aftershaves tone the skin after shaving, help reduce redness and skin irritation, and close the pores. Choosing the essential oils you use in your aftershaves means you can not only customize the fragrance to your preference but you can also choose oils that are helpful for the condition of the skin. For instance, a young man just beginning to shave may have acne or delicate skin, and you can choose essential oils to treat both these skin conditions.

Eye washes and eye compresses provide a wonderful relief for tired, red, or itchy eyes. Regular use of these natural homemade remedies can also help prevent eye conditions, such as conjunctivitis, from arising. It is important to remember that you must never put essential oils near, or in, the eyes themselves. These homemade eye washes and eye compresses use herbal infusions and flower waters rather than essential oils and are gentle enough to use on the eyes.

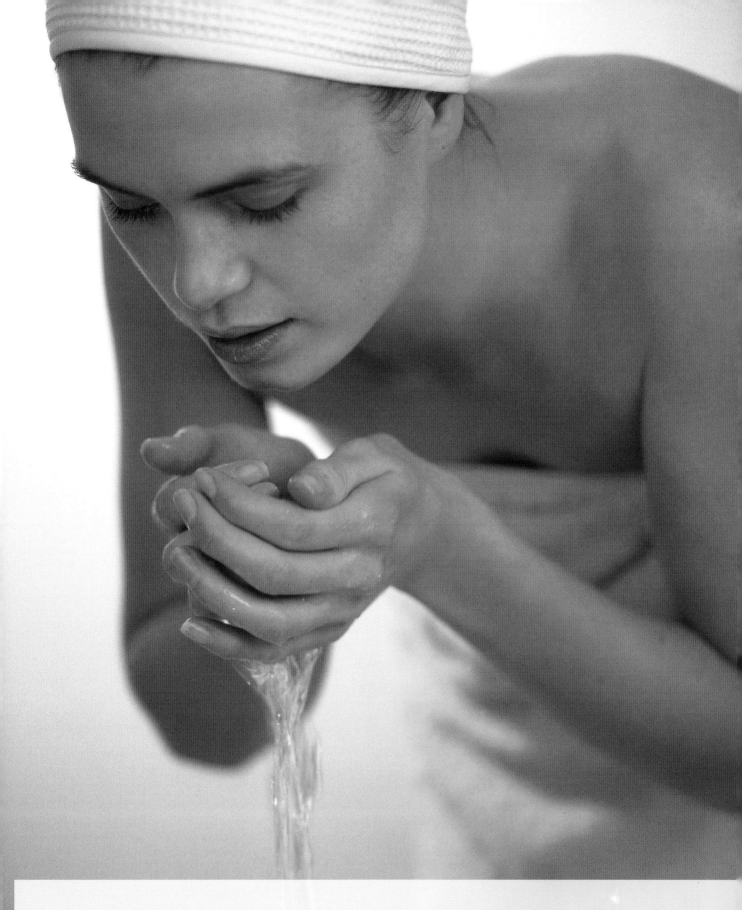

Tip: *Using your homemade deodorants means you may need to wash under your arms a little more frequently, and reapply the deodorant more often—a small price to pay for deodorizing your body naturally.*

Tip: *If you suffer from sweaty feet, you can use this deodorant on your feet as well as under your arms, as the cypress helps prevent excessive sweating.*

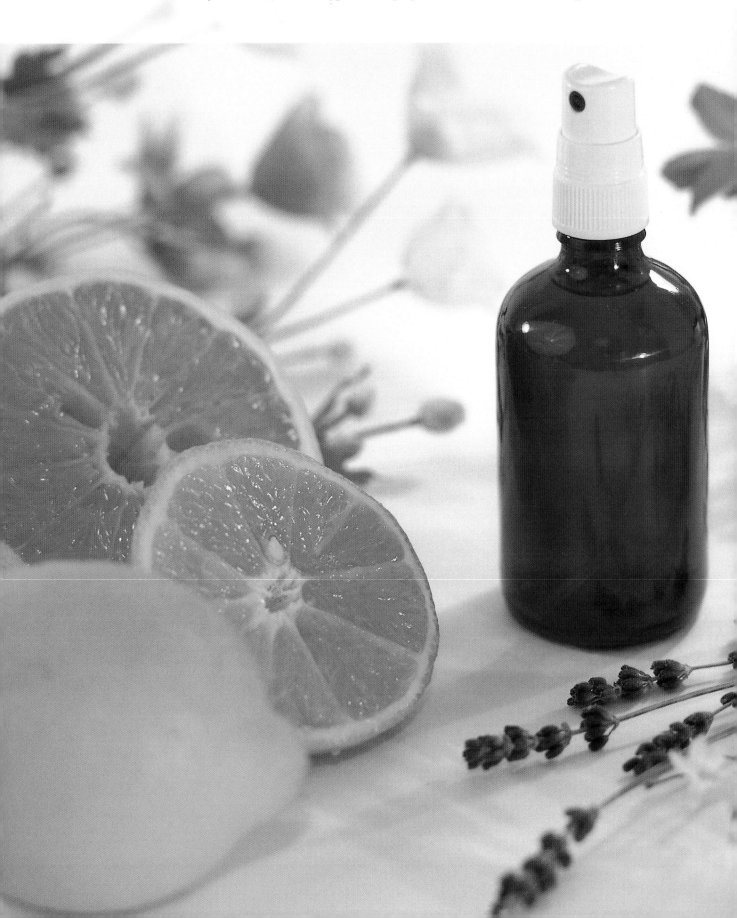

Deodorants

A quick look at the history of deodorants and perfumes reveals that personal hygiene arrived later than the fragrancing of personal objects, such as gloves, bed linens, and clothes. Indeed, until modern sanitary ware was invented, washing was considered a bit of a nuisance rather than the daily necessity we now take for granted.

This means that deodorants and perfumes were used to mask body odors, which is still the role of deodorants today. However, by using the following homemade deodorants, you are only applying natural, plant-based ingredients to your body. These work in harmony with your skin and body, keeping you naturally fresh and clean.

Geranium and Cypress Deodorant

This is a classic combination of essential oils with deodorant properties. Geranium is used in skin-care products for its delightful, sweet floral perfume and its astringent and antiseptic properties. Cypress helps reduce excessive sweating, and its fine, woody smell enhances this deodorant. The classic fragrance is deeply refreshing with hints of floral, citrus, and wood, and is suitable for both women and men.

what's in it?

1 tsp high proof vodka
10 drops geranium
10 drops cypress
8 drops bergamot
5 drops neroli
4 drops lavender
3 drops black pepper
4 tbsp (40 ml) witch hazel
2 tbsp (25 ml) cornflower water
2 tbsp (25 ml) orange flower water

how's it made?

1 Measure the vodka into a 4 oz (100 ml) glass bottle with a spray attachment. Carefully add the essential oils, one by one. Shake vigorously to dissolve the essential oils.

2 Pour the witch hazel into the bottle, using a funnel if necessary, followed by the two flower waters. Shake well.

3 Label the bottle and the deodorant is now ready to use.

4 Before you use the deodorant each time, give the bottle a good shake to ensure the essential oils are fully dispersed.

Citrus and Herbal Deodorant

This gentle, antibacterial deodorant uses some of the most effective deodorant essential oils, including bergamot, thyme, and clary sage. Blended with flower waters and witch hazel into a refreshing spray, this deodorant has a delicious, refreshing aroma that is suitable for both women and men.

what's in it?

1 tsp high proof vodka

10 drops bergamot

8 drops clary sage

7 drops thyme

5 drops rosewood

5 drops lemon

3 drops lavender

2 drops mandarin

4 tbsp (40 ml) witch hazel

2 tbsp (25 ml) linden flower water

2 tbsp (25 ml) orange flower water

how's it made?

1 Measure the vodka into a 4 oz (100 ml) glass bottle with a spray attachment. Carefully add the essential oils, one by one. Shake vigorously to dissolve the essential oils.

2 Pour the witch hazel into the bottle, using a funnel if necessary, followed by the two flower waters. Shake well.

3 Label the bottle and the deodorant is now ready to use.

4 Before you use the deodorant each time, give the bottle a good shake to ensure the essential oils are fully dispersed.

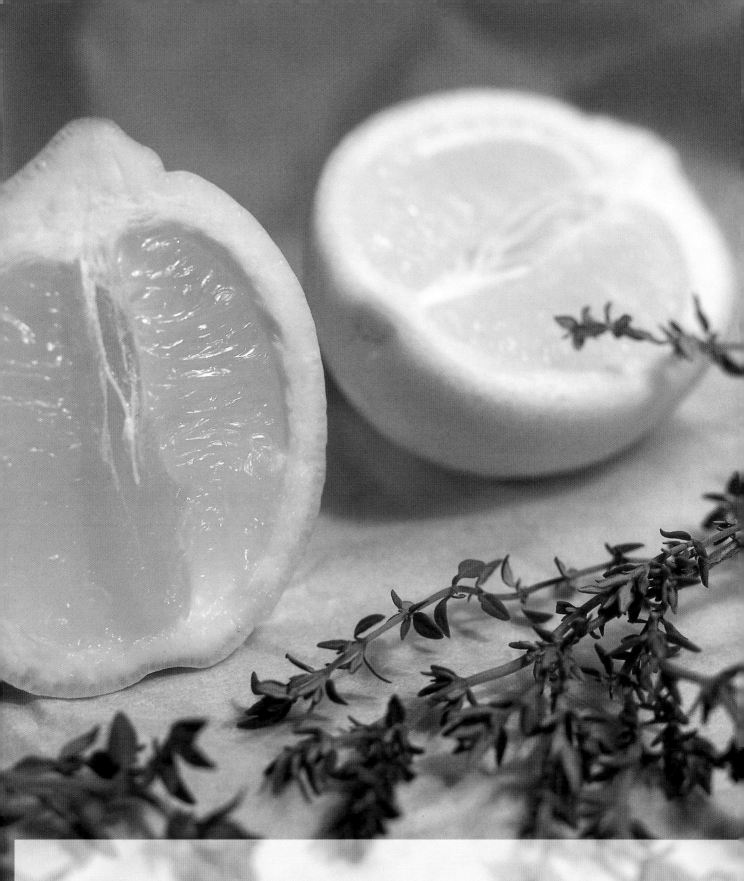

Did You Know? *The ancient Assyrians had a tradition of the men deodorizing their beards.*

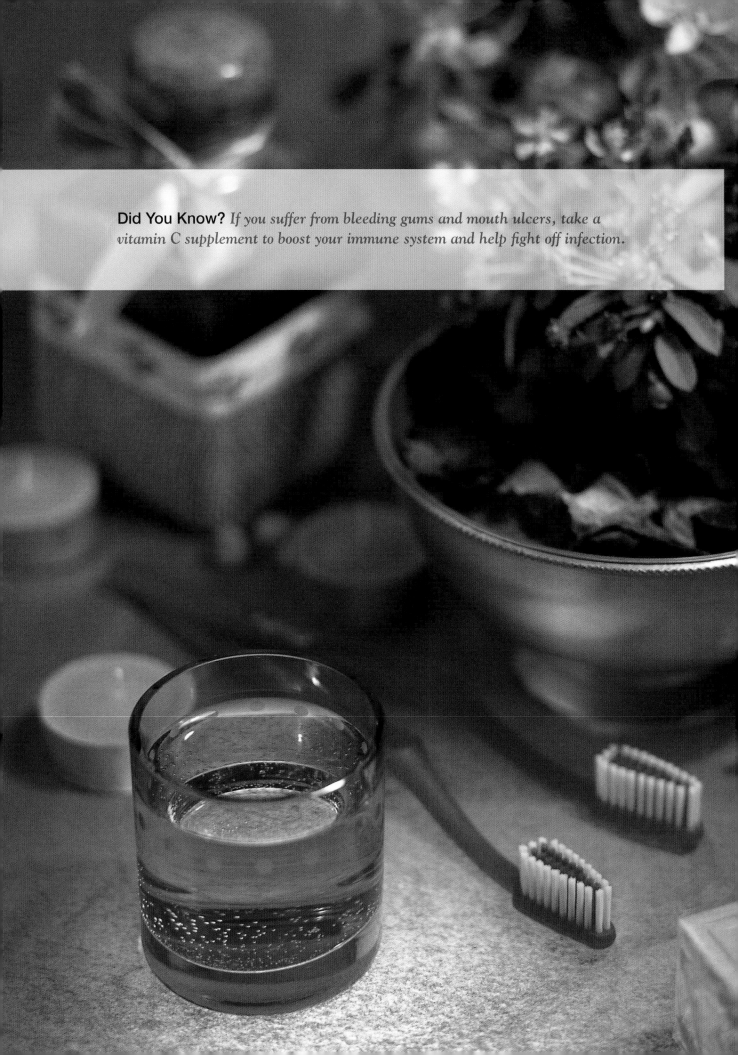

Did You Know? *If you suffer from bleeding gums and mouth ulcers, take a vitamin C supplement to boost your immune system and help fight off infection.*

Mouthwashes

Using a mouthwash daily helps keep your gums healthy and your breath smelling fresh. This daily ritual also helps prevent the build up of plaque on your teeth. Alongside the regular brushing of your teeth with toothpaste and flossing between the teeth, gargles and mouthwashes form an essential part of your daily mouth hygiene routine.

Certain essential oils are very effective in keeping your gums in tip-top condition. Myrrh is traditionally used in toothpastes and mouthwashes as it quickly heals gum disorders and heals mouth ulcers. Fennel is also recommended for use in gargles and mouthwashes as it helps clear gum infections and keeps the mouth smelling fresh and sweet. Alongside peppermint, fennel helps counteract the bitterness of myrrh.

As the following two mouthwashes contain essential oils, remember to spit them out after rinsing your mouth.

Myrrh and Mint Mouthwash

This mouthwash is especially effective if you are having trouble with your gums bleeding or you tend to develop mouth ulcers. The action of the mouthwash is reinforced by using tincture of myrrh as a direct topical application. Put a drop or two of tincture of myrrh on your fingertip and rub over the affected area. It will sting briefly and taste very bitter but the healing effect is well worth it.

what's in it?
6 tbsp (90 ml) high proof brandy or vodka
10 drops myrrh
10 drops peppermint
2 drops lemon
1 drop thyme

how's it made?
1 Pour the brandy or vodka into a 4 oz (100 ml) glass bottle. Carefully add the essential oils one by one. Shake the bottle vigorously to dissolve the oils.

2 Label the bottle and the mouthwash is ready to use. To make one dose of mouthwash, add two or three teaspoons of mouthwash to half a small glass of warm water and stir well.

Fennel Fresh Mouthwash

The clean, fresh, herbal aroma of fennel is balanced with the fruity zing of grapefruit in this tangy mouthwash. Fennel also has a slight aniseed flavor, making it pleasant to use in a mouthwash as well as keeping your mouth and gums clean and healthy.

what's in it?
6 tbsp (90 ml) high proof brandy or vodka

10 drops fennel

10 drops grapefruit

2 drops thyme

1 drop chamomile

how's it made?
1 Pour the brandy or vodka into a 4 oz (100 ml) glass bottle. Carefully add the essential oils, one by one. Shake the bottle vigorously to dissolve the oils.

2 Label the bottle and the mouthwash is ready to use. To make one dose of mouthwash, add two or three teaspoons of mouthwash to half a small glass of warm water and stir well.

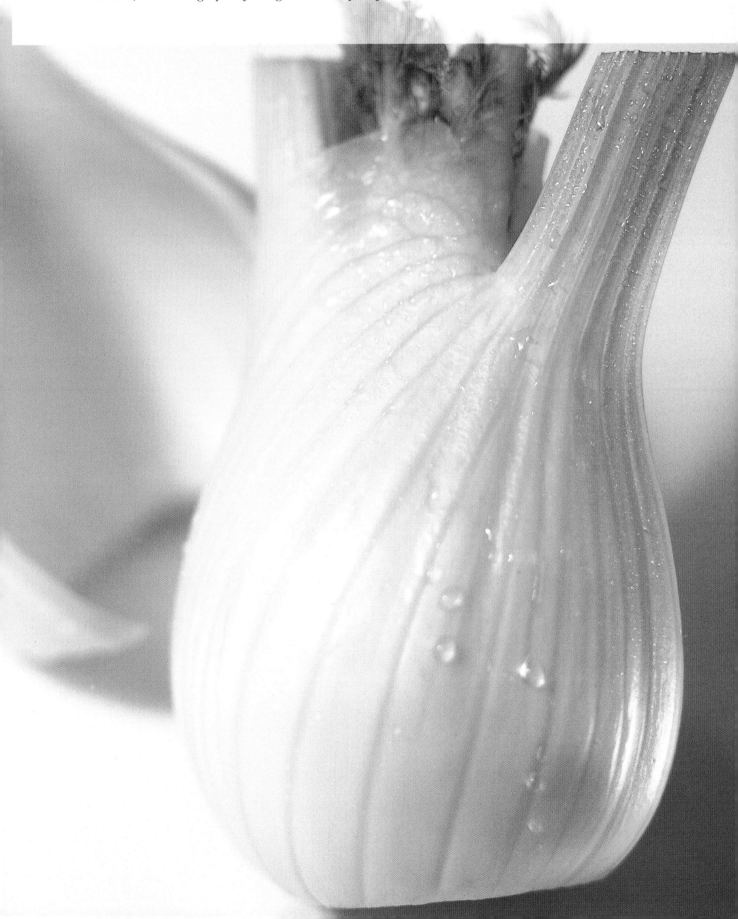

Did You Know? *More people lose their teeth from gum disease than from bad teeth, so looking after your gums is very important.*

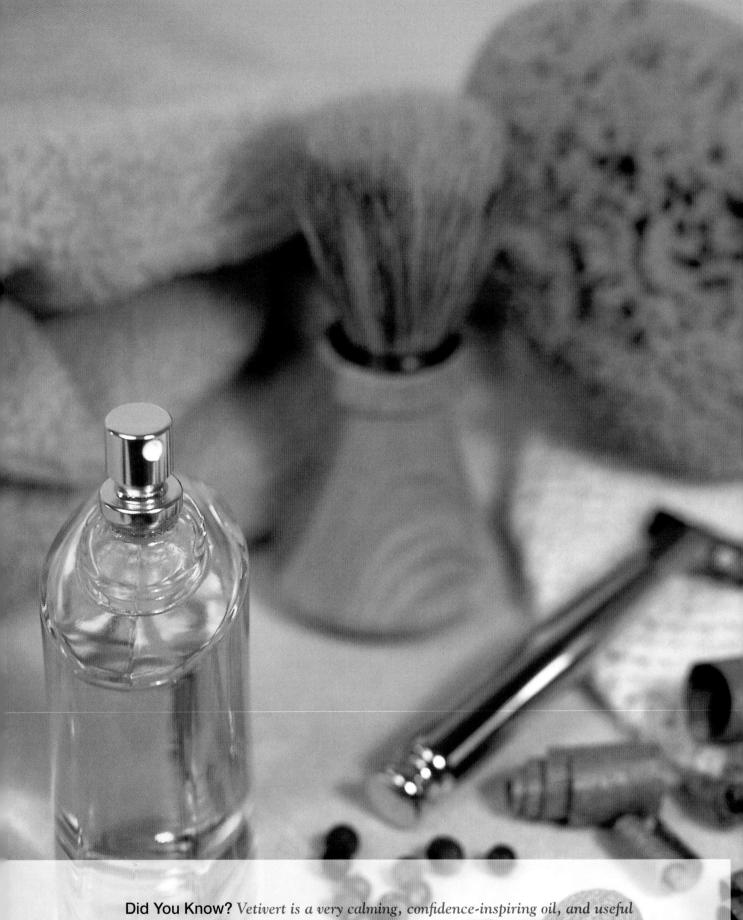

Did You Know? *Vetivert is a very calming, confidence-inspiring oil, and useful for dreamy or overintellectual people.*

Aftershaves

These homemade aftershaves are particularly good for men with sensitive skin and for young men just starting to shave. They are effective but very gentle and help control and prevent razor burn. There are plenty of woody and masculine smelling essential oils that are acceptable to even the most masculine tastes.

Many commercial aftershaves have sickly, cloying, or overpowering scents. The aftershave recipes included here are perfumed only with pure essential oils, and provide more subtle, pleasing, and delicate fragrances. In addition, they tone the skin and close the pores, keeping the skin in good condition.

Sandalwood and Vetivert Aftershave

The sweet, woody, and musky aroma of sandalwood is a particular favorite in aftershaves. Sandalwood is a natural bactericide and soothes the skin after shaving. Vetivert has a deep, earthy aroma that blends beautifully with the sandalwood, creating a strong, deep male fragrance. This aftershave is suitable for all skin types and is particularly good for young men just beginning to shave.

what's in it?
1½ tbsp (20 ml) high proof vodka

8 drops sandalwood

6 drops vetivert

3 drops neroli

4 tbsp (50 ml) witch hazel

6½ tbsp (100 ml) rose water

how's it made?

1 Pour the vodka into a 7 oz (200 ml) glass bottle. Carefully add the essential oils, one by one, and shake vigorously until the oils have dissolved.

2 Add the witch hazel and shake well. Then add the rose water and shake again.

3 Label the bottle and the Sandalwood and Vetivert Aftershave is ready to use.

4 Make sure to shake the bottle before using each time to disperse the oils.

Cedarwood and Juniper Aftershave

Out of all the essential oils, cedarwood is the most popular amongst men, and is much used in men's toiletries. The astringent and antiseptic properties of cedarwood, together with its masculine aroma, make it an obvious choice for a homemade aftershave. Cypress and juniper complement the cedarwood, creating a deep woody fragrance.

what's in it?

1½ tbsp (20 ml) high proof vodka

8 drops cedarwood

6 drops cypress

3 drops juniper

4 tbsp (50 ml) witch hazel

6½ tbsp (100 ml) orange flower water

how's it made?

1 Pour the vodka into a 7 oz (200 ml) glass bottle. Carefully add the essential oils, one by one, and shake vigorously until the oils have dissolved.

2 Add the witch hazel and shake well. Then add the orange flower water and shake again.

3 Label the bottle and the aftershave is ready to use.

4 Make sure to shake the bottle before using each time to disperse the oils.

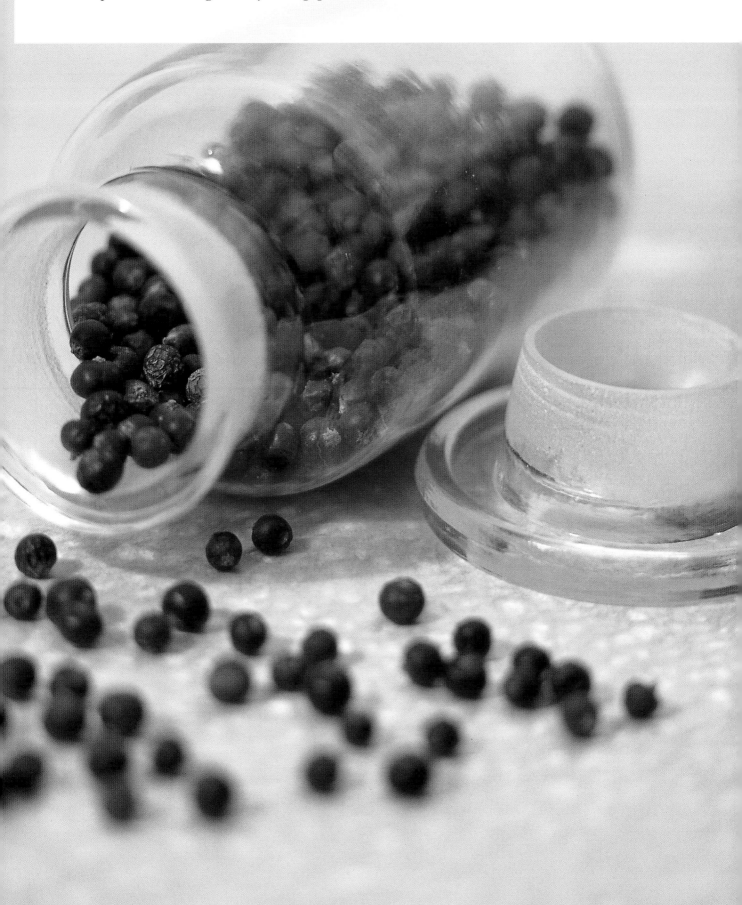

Did You Know? *The popularity of using juniper in men's toiletries is due in part to its cooling and refreshing qualities.*

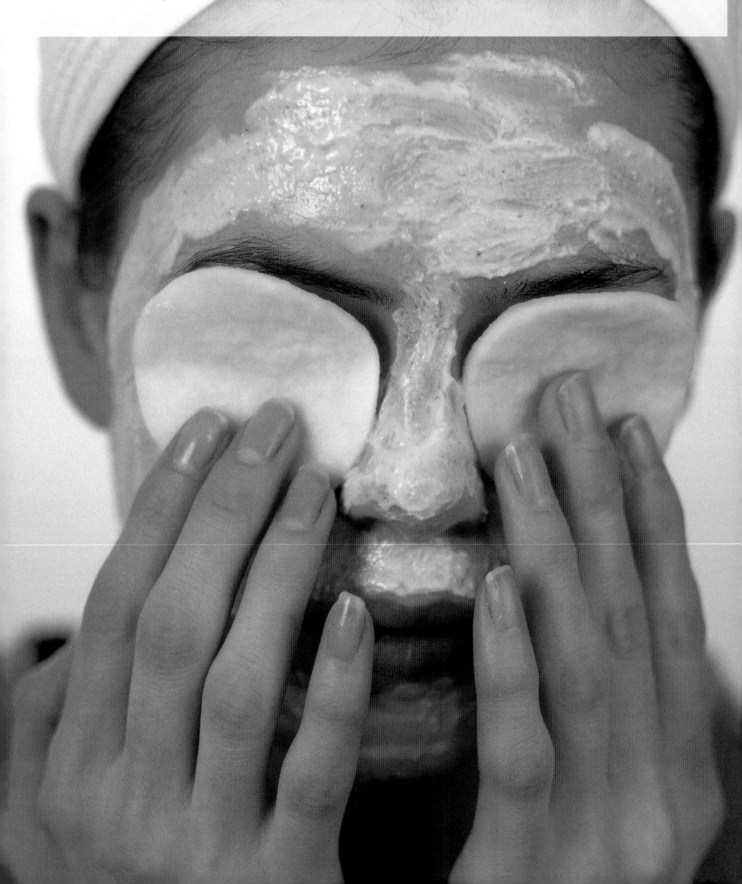

Tip: *Eye infections are very contagious. If you have only one eye that is affected, make sure you use a fresh application of the eyewash on the unaffected eye. In fact, it is good practice to use a fresh application for each eye as a standard procedure.*

Eye Washes and Compresses

Whenever your eyes are tired, red, and itchy, or you have a mild eye infection such as conjunctivitis, then eye washes and eye compresses made from herbal infusions and flower waters can relieve the symptoms naturally. The recipes that follow use easily obtainable ingredients to make simple remedies. However, if you are short of time or desperate, simply washing the eyes with rose water followed by compresses of used, cooled chamomile tea bags can be effective.

An alternative is to use a homeopathic remedy called euphrasia. This is available both as a liquid and as tablets. Use three to four drops of the liquid in cooled boiled water and rinse the eyes with it. Take tablets as recommended by a homeopath.

Chamomile and Eyebright Eye Wash

Using an infusion of organic chamomile blended with cornflower water makes a cooling, refreshing, and healing eye wash. The addition of tincture of eyebright reinforces the healing action, leaving your eyes refreshed and cooled. There is a long tradition of using cornflower water to wash and refresh the eyes.

what's in it?
1 organic chamomile tea bag
Boiling water to infuse the tea bag
1 tbsp (10 ml) cornflower water
4 drops tincture of eyebright

how's it made?

1 Make an infusion of chamomile as you would make an ordinary cup of tea. Leave it to steep for fifteen minutes.

2 Measure out 1 tbsp (10 ml) of chamomile infusion—you can drink the rest of the tea—and pour it into a 1 oz (25 ml) glass bottle.

3 Add the cornflower water and shake well. Add the eyebright tincture and again shake well.

4 The eye wash is ready to use. Wash each eye with approximately half the quantity of eye wash, as you need to make a fresh batch each time.

Rose Water and Elderflower Eye Compresses

These cooling, refreshing eye compresses can be used whenever you have ten or fifteen minutes to rest somewhere quietly with your eyes closed. They are effective for eyes that are stinging as a result of air pollution in cities and built up urban areas. You can use the compresses after an eye wash or on their own.

what's in it?
2 drops tincture of elderflower

1 tbsp (10 ml) rose water

2 cotton pads

how's it made?

1 Carefully pour the tincture of elderflower into a small bottle and top off with the rose water. Shake well.

2 Soak the cotton pads with the mixture, apply to your closed eyes, and lie back and rest for ten or fifteen minutes.

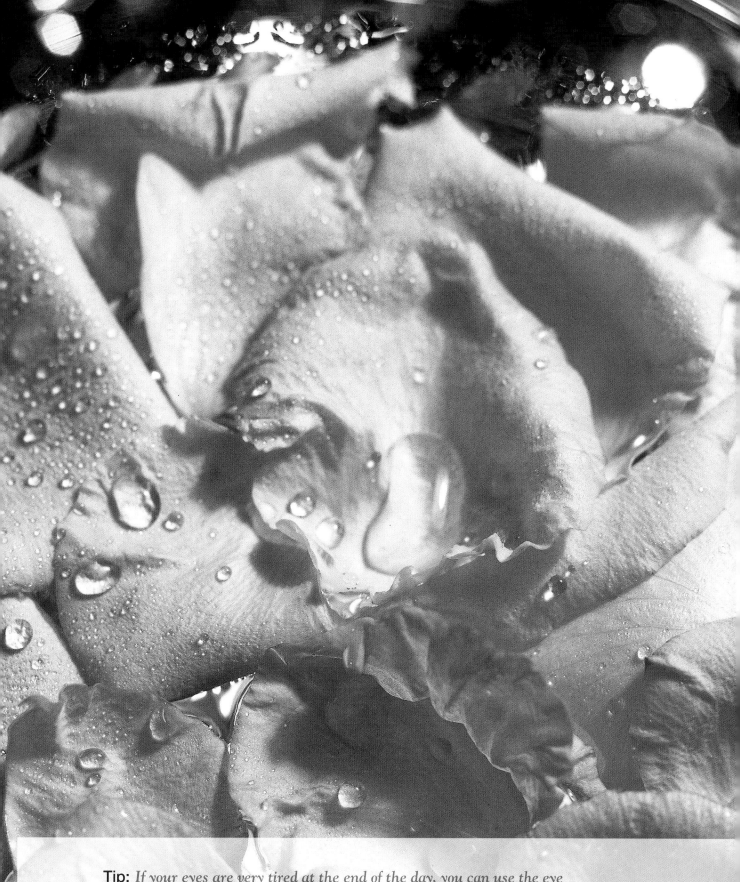

Tip: *If your eyes are very tired at the end of the day, you can use the eye compresses when you go to bed. They will, of course, fall off at some point in the night, but they will have done their work and dried out by then.*

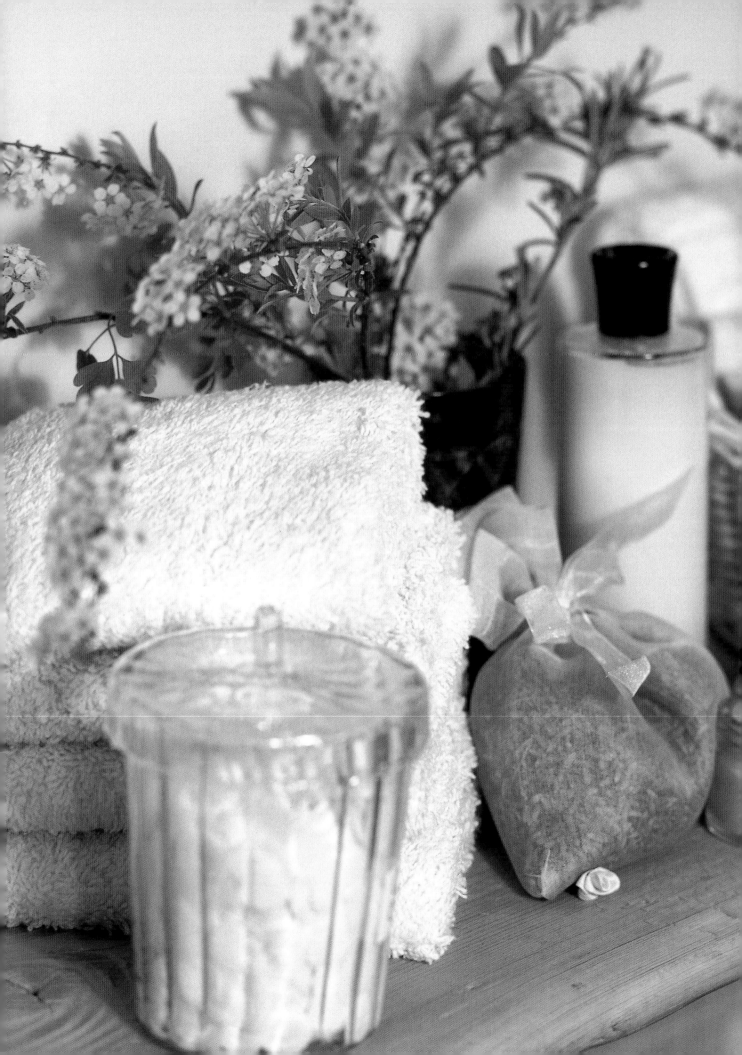

Chapter Seven

Gift Wrapping and Storing Your Cosmetics

How To Present Your Cosmetics

Now that you have created some of these wonderful homemade cosmetics, you need some ideas on storing them well. As they make such lovely gifts, some tips on gift wrapping your different homemade creams, lotions, and so forth are also included.

Once your cosmetics have been made, they should be stored carefully. Because they are made from natural, organic ingredients, they do not contain synthetics nor the chemical preservatives found in many store-bought cosmetics. So, although your homemade cosmetics are nice to use, they will not last as long as their store-bought equivalents. This is why the recipes suggest making up quite small quantities: your creams and toners will be used up long before they start to deteriorate.

Another solution to storing your homemade cosmetics is to give some of them away to friends and family! Natural, organic skin- and hair-care products make wonderful health and beauty enhancing gifts, and using some imaginative packaging and presentation ideas can make them look even more attractive. Some of your homemade cosmetics, such as eye washes and face masks, are made to be used immediately and are, unfortunately, not suitable as gifts.

Many of your creams, lotions, lip balms, toners, and aftershaves are kept in glass jars and bottles. You will have noticed that some of the recipes suggest using dark glass while others indicate that clear glass is fine. If you are making cosmetics to give away as gifts—and even to enjoy yourself—try to purchase attractive glass jars and bottles.

With a little effort, you can find pretty-shaped, decorative clear glass bottles, which look much nicer than the plain variety. The most common dark glass jars and bottles are made from amber glass but these can look a bit boring, or even as if they contain medicinal products. A much more attractive option is to seek out dark blue, dark green, and dark red glass jars and bottles. Silver and gold opaque glass jars are also available, which look quite stunning.

Displaying Your Cosmetics

Although your homemade cosmetics need to be kept out of direct sunlight, displaying them attractively on a shelf or on top of a chest of drawers or dressing table can make an attractive room decoration.

A small pyramid of jars makes an eye catching display. Start with three jars on the bottom layer, then two jars on top of those, and finally one jar at the top. Try mixing different colored jars, such as dark blue and silver for a dramatic look.

Take a selection of bottles of toners and lotions and line them up, mixing colors and heights of the bottles. Take an empty bottle, fill it with water, add a small spray of flowers or a single rosebud, and insert in the middle of the line of bottles.

Place folded dark green or blue hand towels and linens on a bathroom shelf, then add bottles and jars of the same color for a coordinated bathroom display.

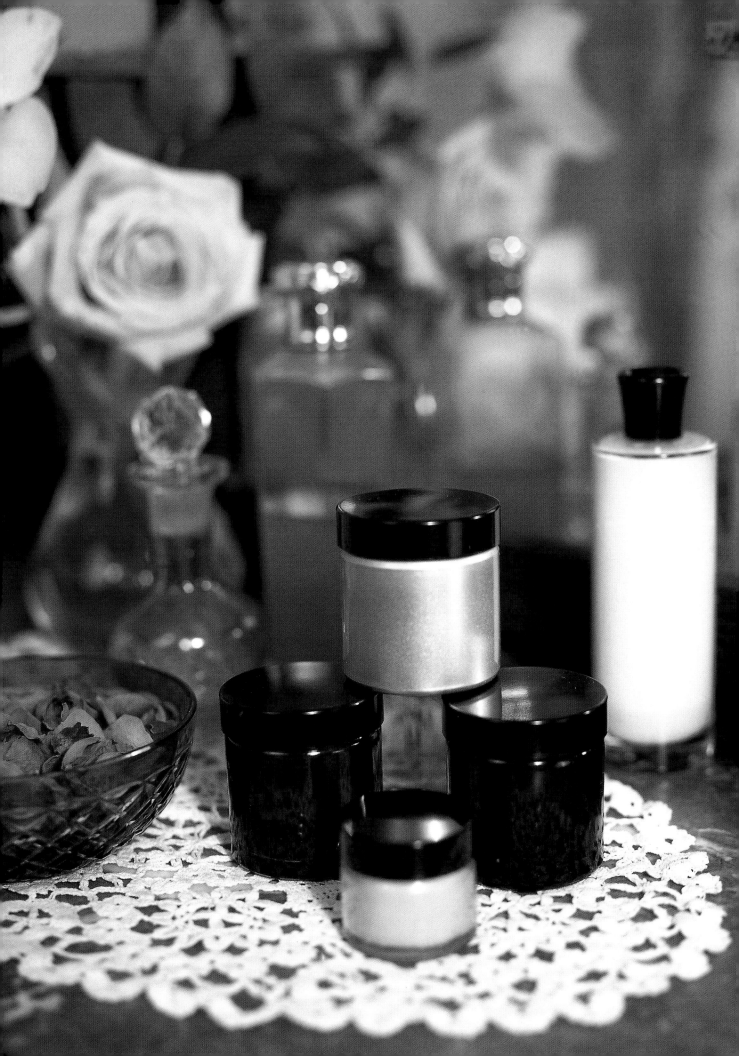

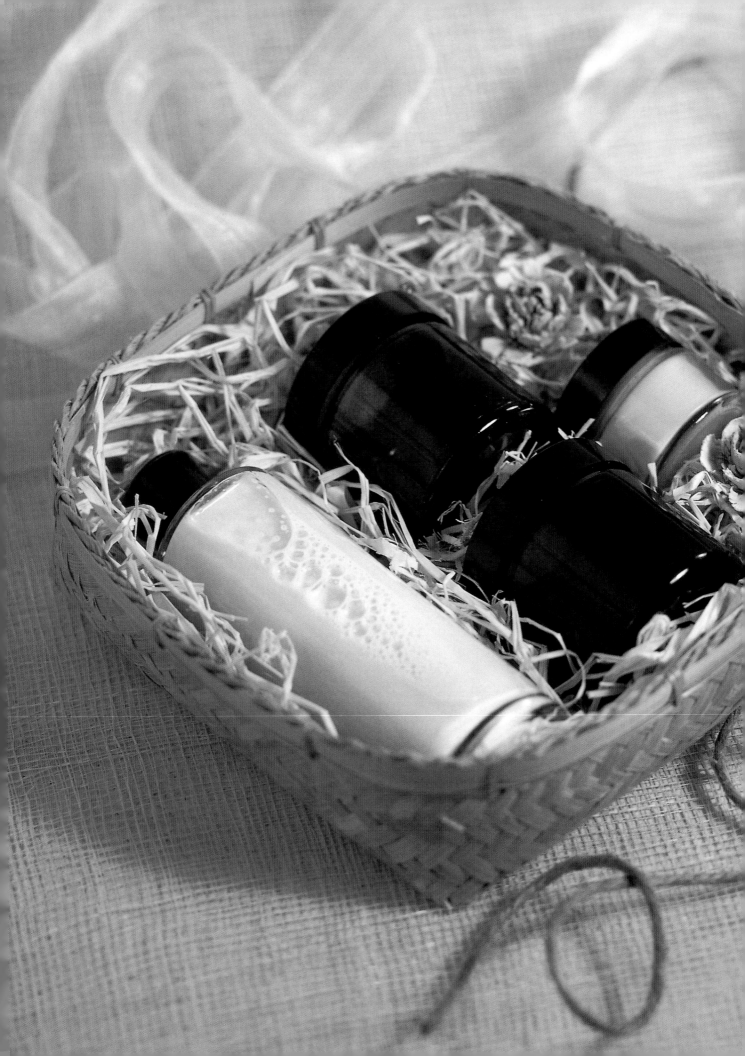

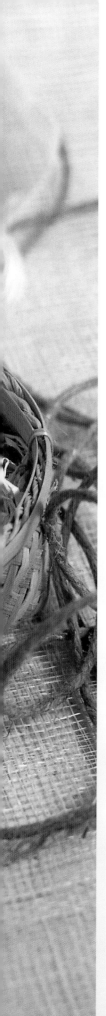

Types of Packaging

Once you have made your lotions and potions, and found attractive glass bottles and jars to put them in, you need to consider how to gift wrap the cosmetics you wish to give away as gifts. The most important point to consider is that glass jars and bottles are fragile, so the packaging must be sturdy enough to protect them adequately and avoid the risk of breakage. Following are some tips for gift wrapping your homemade cosmetics.

Corrugated cardboard is ideal for protecting your jars of face cream and bottles of toner. For bottles, try wrapping a double width length around the bottle twice. Secure with tape, and tie a ribbon, colored string, or strand of raffia around, finishing with a bow. Now fold the open ends closed in a pleat, and either glue them closed or secure them with tape.

Some handcrafted papers are quite stiff and make an attractive alternative to corrugated cardboard. You can fray the ends for a rustic look or cut them with pinking shears.

Colored tissue paper makes an attractive wrapping but is not sufficient on its own to protect glass jars and bottles. Try wrapping a sheet of colored tissue around your jars and bottles, and then wrapping with corrugated cardboard or handcrafted paper.

Boxes—either wood or cardboard—are ideal to package and present your jars and bottles. Try nestling the bottles and jars in shredded paper, raffia, or colored tissue paper. You could also include dried flowers for extra effect.

For a stunning present, take a large wooden box and fill it with a selection of dried flowers and petals. Choose three or four handmade cosmetics that complement each other; a nice combination might include Honey and Rose Lip Balm (page 63), Rose and Geranium skin toner (page 35), Cocoa Butter and Rose Cream (page 47), and Rejuvenating Rose Bath Milk (page 74). Place the different bottles and jars in among the dried flowers and wrap a sheet of clear plastic over the top.

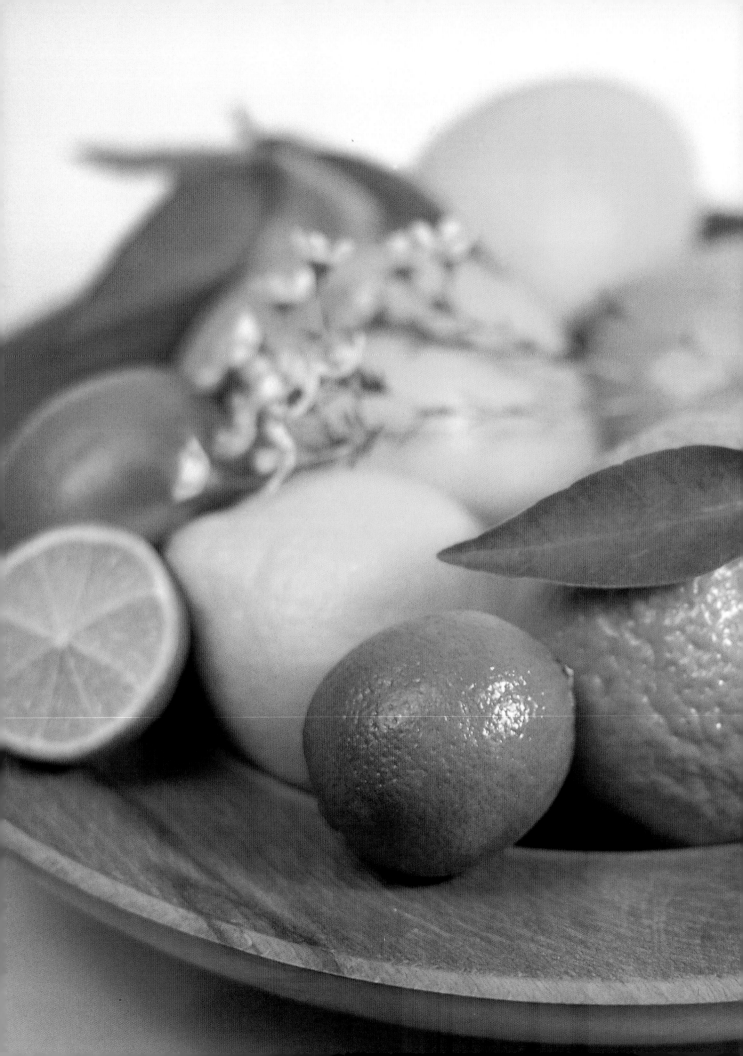

Chapter Eight

Buying and Storing Fresh and Dried Ingredients

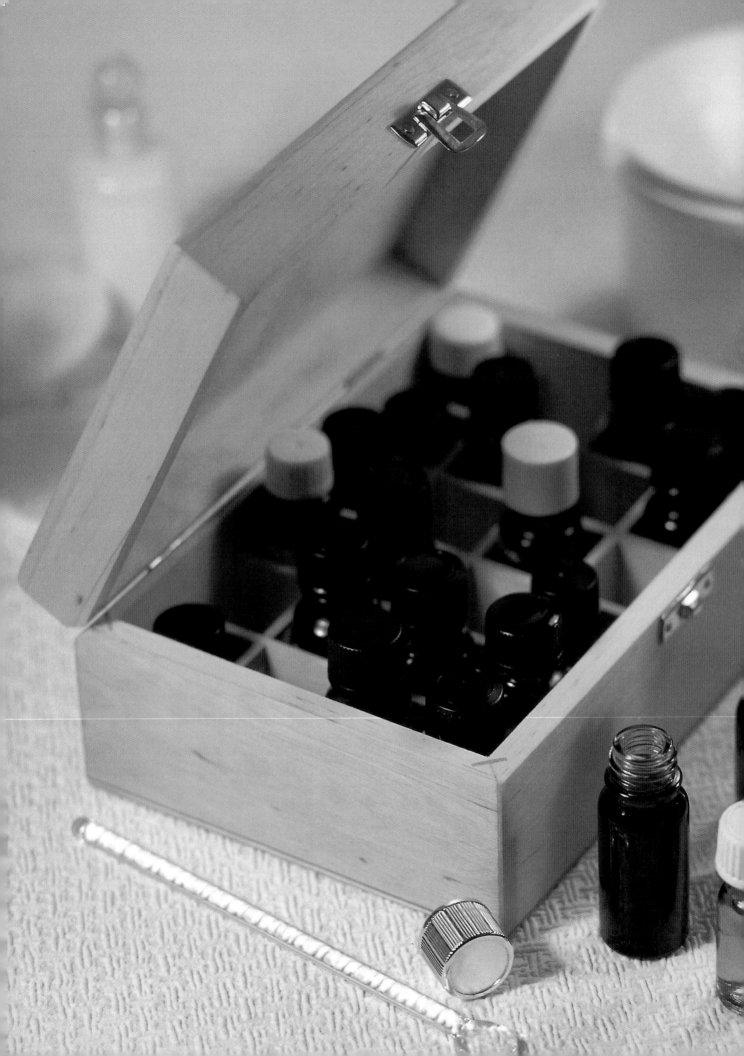

Storing Fresh and Dried Ingredients

Buying and storing all your homemade cosmetic ingredients properly is of fundamental importance to the overall process of making them. The suppliers listed in the directory on the following two pages give you a range of professional suppliers of all the ingredients you will need to successfully make skin creams, lotions, toners, deodorants, shampoos, conditioners, and so forth. Following are some tips on how to store and keep your ingredients properly, and also tips on storing your skin-care products once you've made them.

- All ingredients are best bought fresh. Although the different ingredients for the various cosmetics have differing shelf lives, it is a good habit to buy your ingredients only as you need them.

- Only buy sufficient quantities for your immediate requirements. Even if you can receive a discount for buying larger quantities of ingredients, unless you use it up quickly it could prove a false economy.

- Store your ingredients in a cool, dark, dry place away from drafts, light, damp, and heat. This will help prolong shelf life.

- Make sure you store your bottles of essential oils upright, in a cool dark place.

- Many flower waters are supplied in thick, clear plastic bottles. Transfer them into dark glass bottles as soon as possible. Flower waters only have a limited shelf life, and storing them in dark glass bottles will help prolong this somewhat.

- Fresh ingredients such as yogurt, ground almonds, cucumber, herbs, fruits, and honey should be as fresh as possible, especially for organic produce.

- If you have used half a container of base lotion, cleanser, skin cream, or other base product, consider transferring the remainder to a smaller container. This will prevent too much air from coming into contact with the base ingredient, which could spoil it more rapidly.

- If you think something has gone bad because it has discolored or changed texture, then throw it away and buy new supplies. Using old, imperfect ingredients could affect how a recipe turns out, and you don't want to waste other ingredients.

Suppliers of Ingredients in the USA and UK

Suppliers in the USA

Alban Muller International
Distributed in USA by
Tri-K Industries
27 Bland Street
P. O. Box 312
Emerson, NJ 07630
(201) 261-2800

Aphrodisia Products Inc.
62 Kent Street
Brooklyn, NY 11222
(718) 383-3677

The Essence of Life
502 Camino Cortez
Taos, NM 87571
(505) 758-7941
info@newmex.com

Essential Oil Company
1719 Southeast Umatilla Street
Portland, OR 97202
(800) 729-5912
order@essentialoil.com

Fragrant Earth
2000 2nd Avenue, Suite 206
Seattle, WA 98121
(206) 374-9020
jade@theida.com

Janca's Jojoba Oil & Seed Co
456 East Juanita, #7
Mesa, AZ 85204
(602) 497-11125

Prima Fleur Botanicals Inc
12,01-R Andersen Drive
San Rafael, CA 94901
(415) 455-0957

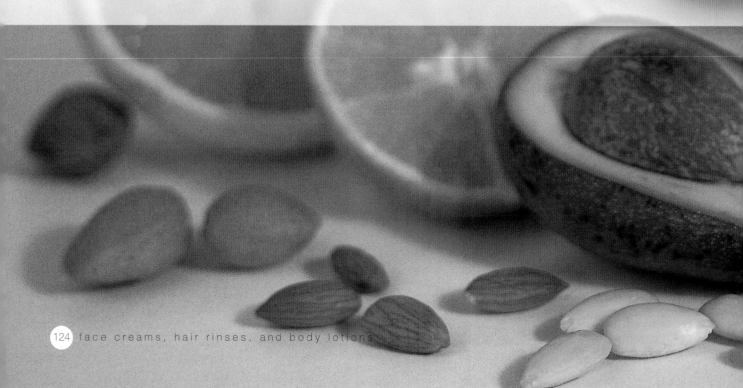

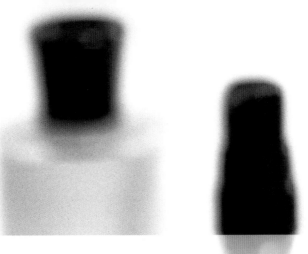

Suppliers in the UK

G Baldwin & Co
173 Walworth Road
London SE17 1RW
(020) 7252 6264
sales@baldwins.co.uk

Butterbur & Sage
7 Tessa Road
Reading
Berkshire RG1 8HH
(0118) 950 5100
butterburandsage@btinternet.com

Essentially Oils
8–10 Mount Farm Junction Road
Churchill Chipping Norton
Oxfordshire OX7 6NP
(01608) 659 544
sales@essentiallyoils.com

Fragrant Earth Co Ltd
Orchard Court Magdalene Street
Glastonbury Somerset BA6 9 EW
(01458) 831 361
all-enquiries@fragrant-earth.com

Nature's Treasures
Bridge Industrial Estate
New Portreath Road Bridge
Near Redruth
Cornwall TR16 4QL
(01209) 843 881
naturestreasures@ndirect.co.uk

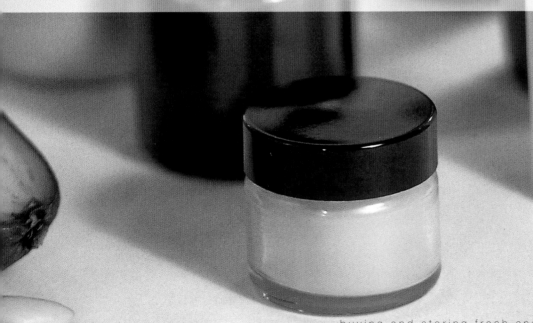